the
integrative nutrition
journal

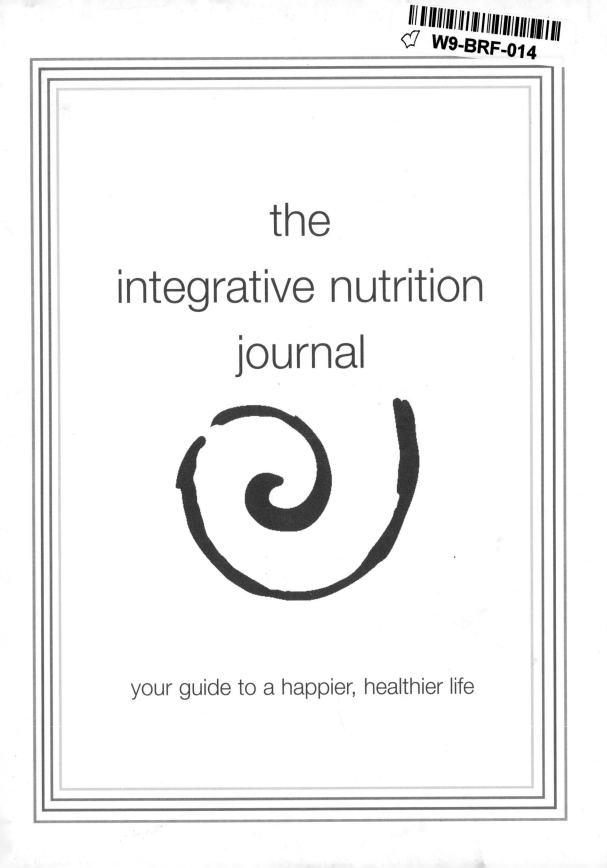

your guide to a happier, healthier life

ISBN 0-9773025-1-2

Published by Integrative Nutrition Publishing, Inc.
3 East 28 Street
New York, NY 10016
www.integrativenutrition.com

Special thanks to Robin Peglow
for inspiring and co-creating this journal with us.

Robin Peglow Berg
SOUL Moxie coaching
www.soulmoxie.net
303-282-1077

All quotes are from members of Integrative Nutrition's distinguished faculty.

Printed on recycled paper.

introduction

At Integrative Nutrition, we are creating the future of nutrition by encouraging, cultivating and promoting healthy eating and balanced living. We are dedicated to inspiring all people to live happy, healthy lives, including you. It is extremely important for you to be well. Without good health, you cannot live the incredible life you were born to live.

Understanding what and how to eat is essential for wellness. You are walking food. The food you take into your mouth gets assimilated into your bloodstream. Your blood is what creates your cells, your tissues, your organs, your skin, your hair, your brain, and eventually, your thoughts and feelings. People who eat high-quality, nutritious foods naturally have higher energy, stronger digestion and clearer thinking than those who eat fast foods or junk foods. Wherever you fall on this spectrum is completely okay. But now that you have this book, your life and your health are only going to get better.

Your body is completely intelligent. It is constantly sending you messages about what it needs for health and balance. These messages appear as cravings, intuitions and, sometimes, health problems. This book will teach you to listen to your body's wisdom, deconstruct your health concerns and choose the foods you need for vibrant health.

Beyond food, other forms of nourishment—what our school calls primary food— are essential for health. A spiritual practice, a desired career, regular physical activity and healthy relationships fill your soul and satisfy your hunger for living. When primary food is balanced and fulfilling, the fun, excitement and passion of your daily life feed you, making what you eat secondary.

This journal is designed to guide and support you as you discover the primary and secondary foods that are right for you. Use it with the intention of permanently changing your relationship to food and health, because it will.

This approach is not about acquiring
more self-discipline or willpower.
It's about personally discovering what
nourishes you, what feeds you and
ultimately what makes your life extraordinary.

Joshua Rosenthal, MScEd, Founder and Director,
Institute for Integrative Nutrition

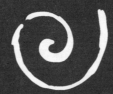

how to use this journal

Be Yourself
You are an individual with your own unique schedule and style. We've designed this book as a three-month daily journal, but use it however you choose—once a day, twice a week, whatever works for you. Practice being your own authority on your life and health. Your body has all the answers you need. Be honest with yourself and trust that the little changes you make over time will lead to huge transformation. Relax, have fun and be yourself.

Morning Intentions
Begin each day in a positive way, checking in with yourself and expressing gratitude. Then plan out your goals and action steps.

Evening Reflections
Reflect on how your day went. What worked and what did not? Remember to be loving and appreciative of your efforts.

Weekly Check-ins & Guided Exercises
Record your new discoveries and accomplishments. Take time out to brainstorm, doodle and let your creativity flow with the guided exercises.

Monthly Activities & Progress
Complete the Circle of Life and Wish List to clarify your goals and desires. At the end of the month, record and appreciate your great progress. Color coding shows you where to begin and end each month.

If you have questions about any of the terms used in this journal, please see the glossary at the back of the book.

Journaling or expressive writing is a
simple, gentle, and inexpensive
healing technique. I consider it a powerful
therapeutic tool to learn more about yourself
and become aware of how your mind and
emotions can influence you physically.

Andrew Weil, MD

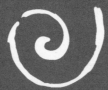

month one

circle of life

This exercise will help you discover which primary foods need attention in order for you to create more balance in your life. The circle has twelve sections. Place a dot on the line for each section to designate how satisfied you are with that aspect of your life. A dot placed towards the center of the circle indicates dissatisfaction, while a dot placed towards the periphery indicates ultimate happiness. When you have placed a dot on each line, connect the dots to see your Circle of Life. Now you have a clear visual of any areas that may need your attention. You will complete this exercise again next month to see if your circle has become more balanced.

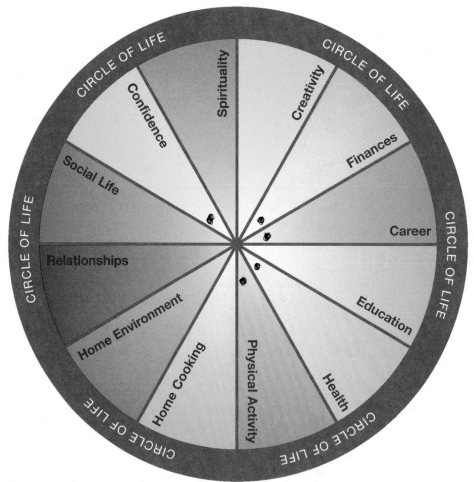

wish list

Now that you have identified areas of your life that are out of balance or unsatisfying, what would it take to bring them into balance? What experiences, items, relationships or feelings would make those parts of your life juicy and exciting? This exercise will help you get in touch with your desires. In the table below, begin listing simple and obvious wishes. Bigger, more exciting desires will come as you write.

Keep these desires in mind when setting your morning intentions. Whenever you fulfill a desire, put an X in the "done" column. In the "gratitude" column, thank anyone who may have helped. You might be thanking yourself. Notice how, as you take better care of yourself, your desires naturally come true, and your life becomes more fulfilling.

	wish	done	gratitude
1	↓ quantity of food eat		
2	lose 25#		
3	↑ flow of income ($)		
4	Insomnia to resolve		
5	↑ exercise significantly		
6	↑ meticulous self care		
7	A very successful practice		
8	↑ self confidence		
9	Continue to have health improve		
10			
11			
12			

morning intentions

date: _1/27/10_

morning thoughts, feelings & intuitions: _____

_____

_____

_____

i am grateful for: _____

_____

_____

_____

goals for today:

○ _Take in ↑ water_____

○ _Watch quantities of food eaten_____

○ _____

action steps for each goal:

○ _____ ○ _____ ○ _____

○ _____ ○ _____ ○ _____

○ _____ ○ _____ ○ _____

fun, relaxation & adventure for today:

○ _____

○ _____

○ _____

evening reflections

- ○ morning intentions
- ○ home-cooked food (__x)
- ○ mindful eating
- ○ reduced one food
- ○ tongue scraper
- ○ hot towel scrub

- ○ hot water bottle
- ○ conscious breathing
- ○ fresh air
- ○ physical activity
- ○ prayer/meditation
- ○ meaningful connections

- ○ loving work
- ○ touch/massage
- ○ laughter
- ○ time to myself
- ○ visualized my future
- ○ quality sleep

high quality nourishment

water/hydrating liquids: _____

whole grains: _____

vegetables: _____

fruits: _____

healthy fats: _____

protein: _____

supplements: _____

how i felt today

mood: _____ digestion: _____

energy: _____ cravings: _____

today i appreciate myself for: _____

_____

choices that did not serve me or support me: _____

_____

today i added in or crowded out: _____

_____

loving thought before bed: _____

_____

morning intentions

date: _____

morning thoughts, feelings & intuitions: _____

_____

_____

_____

i am grateful for: _____

_____

_____

_____

goals for today:

○ _____

○ _____

○ _____

action steps for each goal:

○ _____ ○ _____ ○ _____

○ _____ ○ _____ ○ _____

○ _____ ○ _____ ○ _____

fun, relaxation & adventure for today:

○ _____

○ _____

○ _____

evening reflections

○ morning intentions
○ home-cooked food (__x)
○ mindful eating
○ reduced one food
○ tongue scraper
○ hot towel scrub

○ hot water bottle
○ conscious breathing
○ fresh air
○ physical activity
○ prayer/meditation
○ meaningful connections

○ loving work
○ touch/massage
○ laughter
○ time to myself
○ visualized my future
○ quality sleep

high quality nourishment

water/hydrating liquids: _____

whole grains: _____

vegetables: _____

fruits: _____

healthy fats: _____

protein: _____

supplements: _____

how i felt today

mood: _____ digestion: _____

energy: _____ cravings: _____

today i appreciate myself for: _____

_____

choices that did not serve me or support me: _____

_____

today i added in or crowded out: _____

_____

loving thought before bed: _____

_____

morning intentions

date: _____

morning thoughts, feelings & intuitions: _____

_____

_____

_____

i am grateful for: _____

_____

_____

_____

goals for today:

○ _____

○ _____

○ _____

action steps for each goal:

○ _____ ○ _____ ○ _____

○ _____ ○ _____ ○ _____

○ _____ ○ _____ ○ _____

fun, relaxation & adventure for today:

○ _____

○ _____

○ _____

evening reflections

○ morning intentions
○ home-cooked food (__x)
○ mindful eating
○ reduced one food
○ tongue scraper
○ hot towel scrub

○ hot water bottle
○ conscious breathing
○ fresh air
○ physical activity
○ prayer/meditation
○ meaningful connections

○ loving work
○ touch/massage
○ laughter
○ time to myself
○ visualized my future
○ quality sleep

high quality nourishment

water/hydrating liquids: _____

whole grains: _____

vegetables: _____

fruits: _____

healthy fats: _____

protein: _____

supplements: _____

how i felt today

mood: _____ digestion: _____

energy: _____ cravings: _____

today i appreciate myself for: _____

_____

choices that did not serve me or support me: _____

_____

today i added in or crowded out: _____

_____

loving thought before bed: _____

_____

morning intentions

date: _____

morning thoughts, feelings & intuitions: _____

_____

_____

_____

i am grateful for: _____

_____

_____

_____

goals for today:

O _____

O _____

O _____

action steps for each goal:

O _____ O _____ O _____

O _____ O _____ O _____

O _____ O _____ O _____

fun, relaxation & adventure for today:

O _____

O _____

O _____

evening reflections

- ○ morning intentions
- ○ home-cooked food (__x)
- ○ mindful eating
- ○ reduced one food
- ○ tongue scraper
- ○ hot towel scrub

- ○ hot water bottle
- ○ conscious breathing
- ○ fresh air
- ○ physical activity
- ○ prayer/meditation
- ○ meaningful connections

- ○ loving work
- ○ touch/massage
- ○ laughter
- ○ time to myself
- ○ visualized my future
- ○ quality sleep

high quality nourishment

water/hydrating liquids: _____

whole grains: _____

vegetables: _____

fruits: _____

healthy fats: _____

protein: _____

supplements: _____

how i felt today

mood: _____   digestion: _____

energy: _____   cravings: _____

today i appreciate myself for: _____

_____

choices that did not serve me or support me: _____

_____

today i added in or crowded out: _____

_____

loving thought before bed: _____

_____

morning intentions

date: _____

morning thoughts, feelings & intuitions: _____

_____

_____

_____

i am grateful for: _____

_____

_____

_____

goals for today:

○ _____

○ _____

○ _____

action steps for each goal:

○ _____ ○ _____ ○ _____

○ _____ ○ _____ ○ _____

○ _____ ○ _____ ○ _____

fun, relaxation & adventure for today:

○ _____

○ _____

○ _____

evening reflections

- ○ morning intentions
- ○ home-cooked food (__x)
- ○ mindful eating
- ○ reduced one food
- ○ tongue scraper
- ○ hot towel scrub

- ○ hot water bottle
- ○ conscious breathing
- ○ fresh air
- ○ physical activity
- ○ prayer/meditation
- ○ meaningful connections

- ○ loving work
- ○ touch/massage
- ○ laughter
- ○ time to myself
- ○ visualized my future
- ○ quality sleep

high quality nourishment

water/hydrating liquids: _____

whole grains: _____

vegetables: _____

fruits: _____

healthy fats: _____

protein: _____

supplements: _____

how i felt today

mood: _____   digestion: _____

energy: _____   cravings: _____

today i appreciate myself for: _____

_____

choices that did not serve me or support me: _____

_____

today i added in or crowded out: _____

_____

loving thought before bed: _____

_____

morning intentions

date: _____

morning thoughts, feelings & intuitions: _____
_____
_____
_____

i am grateful for: _____
_____
_____
_____

goals for today:

◯ _____
◯ _____
◯ _____

action steps for each goal:

◯ _____ ◯ _____ ◯ _____
◯ _____ ◯ _____ ◯ _____
◯ _____ ◯ _____ ◯ _____

fun, relaxation & adventure for today:

◯ _____
◯ _____
◯ _____

evening reflections

- ○ morning intentions
- ○ home-cooked food (__x)
- ○ mindful eating
- ○ reduced one food
- ○ tongue scraper
- ○ hot towel scrub

- ○ hot water bottle
- ○ conscious breathing
- ○ fresh air
- ○ physical activity
- ○ prayer/meditation
- ○ meaningful connections

- ○ loving work
- ○ touch/massage
- ○ laughter
- ○ time to myself
- ○ visualized my future
- ○ quality sleep

high quality nourishment

water/hydrating liquids: _____

whole grains: _____

vegetables: _____

fruits: _____

healthy fats: _____

protein: _____

supplements: _____

how i felt today

mood: _____   digestion: _____

energy: _____   cravings: _____

today i appreciate myself for: _____

_____

choices that did not serve me or support me: _____

_____

today i added in or crowded out: _____

_____

loving thought before bed: _____

_____

morning intentions

date: _____

morning thoughts, feelings & intuitions: _____

_____

_____

_____

i am grateful for: _____

_____

_____

_____

goals for today:

○ _____

○ _____

○ _____

action steps for each goal:

○ _____ ○ _____ ○ _____

○ _____ ○ _____ ○ _____

○ _____ ○ _____ ○ _____

fun, relaxation & adventure for today:

○ _____

○ _____

○ _____

evening reflections

- ○ morning intentions
- ○ home-cooked food (__x)
- ○ mindful eating
- ○ reduced one food
- ○ tongue scraper
- ○ hot towel scrub

- ○ hot water bottle
- ○ conscious breathing
- ○ fresh air
- ○ physical activity
- ○ prayer/meditation
- ○ meaningful connections

- ○ loving work
- ○ touch/massage
- ○ laughter
- ○ time to myself
- ○ visualized my future
- ○ quality sleep

high quality nourishment

water/hydrating liquids: _____

whole grains: _____

vegetables: _____

fruits: _____

healthy fats: _____

protein: _____

supplements: _____

how i felt today

mood: _____   digestion: _____

energy: _____   cravings: _____

today i appreciate myself for: _____

_____

choices that did not serve me or support me: _____

_____

today i added in or crowded out: _____

_____

loving thought before bed: _____

_____

weekly check-in

dates: _____

what's new & good?

energy & vitality: _____
_____

chewing & digestion: _____
_____

cravings & addictions: _____
_____

hair & skin: _____
_____

mouth, teeth & tongue: _____
_____

body shape & weight: _____
_____

posture & breathing: _____
_____

mood & emotions: _____
_____

relating to others: _____
_____

about the week

most nourishing food: _____

_____

best primary food: _____

_____

special person i appreciate: _____

_____

biggest challenge: _____

_____

main health concern: _____

_____

greatest accomplishment: _____

_____

most fun i had: _____

_____

i got clear that i really want to: _____

_____

other thoughts: _____

_____

next week I plan to: _____

_____

guided exercise

childhood dreams

What did you want to be when you grew up?

What adventures did you imagine having?

What were your childhood dreams and aspirations?

I never had any

Happiness leads to conditions that tend to bring more happiness.
The more we flourish, the more we are likely to flourish.

James Pawelski, PhD

morning intentions

date: _____

morning thoughts, feelings & intuitions: _____

_____

_____

_____

i am grateful for: _____

_____

_____

_____

goals for today:

○ _____

○ _____

○ _____

action steps for each goal:

○ _____ ○ _____ ○ _____

○ _____ ○ _____ ○ _____

○ _____ ○ _____ ○ _____

fun, relaxation & adventure for today:

○ _____

○ _____

○ _____

evening reflections

- ○ morning intentions
- ○ home-cooked food (__x)
- ○ mindful eating
- ○ reduced one food
- ○ tongue scraper
- ○ hot towel scrub

- ○ hot water bottle
- ○ conscious breathing
- ○ fresh air
- ○ physical activity
- ○ prayer/meditation
- ○ meaningful connections

- ○ loving work
- ○ touch/massage
- ○ laughter
- ○ time to myself
- ○ visualized my future
- ○ quality sleep

high quality nourishment

water/hydrating liquids: _____

whole grains: _____

vegetables: _____

fruits: _____

healthy fats: _____

protein: _____

supplements: _____

how i felt today

mood: _____ digestion: _____

energy: _____ cravings: _____

today i appreciate myself for: _____

_____

choices that did not serve me or support me: _____

_____

today i added in or crowded out: _____

_____

loving thought before bed: _____

_____

morning intentions

date: _____

morning thoughts, feelings & intuitions: _____

_____

_____

_____

i am grateful for: _____

_____

_____

_____

goals for today:

○ _____

○ _____

○ _____

action steps for each goal:

○ _____ ○ _____ ○ _____

○ _____ ○ _____ ○ _____

○ _____ ○ _____ ○ _____

fun, relaxation & adventure for today:

○ _____

○ _____

○ _____

evening reflections

- ○ morning intentions
- ○ home-cooked food (__x)
- ○ mindful eating
- ○ reduced one food
- ○ tongue scraper
- ○ hot towel scrub

- ○ hot water bottle
- ○ conscious breathing
- ○ fresh air
- ○ physical activity
- ○ prayer/meditation
- ○ meaningful connections

- ○ loving work
- ○ touch/massage
- ○ laughter
- ○ time to myself
- ○ visualized my future
- ○ quality sleep

high quality nourishment

water/hydrating liquids: _____

whole grains: _____

vegetables: _____

fruits: _____

healthy fats: _____

protein: _____

supplements: _____

how i felt today

mood: _____ digestion: _____

energy: _____ cravings: _____

today i appreciate myself for: _____

_____

choices that did not serve me or support me: _____

_____

today i added in or crowded out: _____

_____

loving thought before bed: _____

_____

morning intentions

date: _____

morning thoughts, feelings & intuitions: _____

_____

_____

_____

i am grateful for: _____

_____

_____

_____

goals for today:

◯ _____

◯ _____

◯ _____

action steps for each goal:

◯ _____ ◯ _____ ◯ _____

◯ _____ ◯ _____ ◯ _____

◯ _____ ◯ _____ ◯ _____

fun, relaxation & adventure for today:

◯ _____

◯ _____

◯ _____

evening reflections

- ○ morning intentions
- ○ home-cooked food (__x)
- ○ mindful eating
- ○ reduced one food
- ○ tongue scraper
- ○ hot towel scrub

- ○ hot water bottle
- ○ conscious breathing
- ○ fresh air
- ○ physical activity
- ○ prayer/meditation
- ○ meaningful connections

- ○ loving work
- ○ touch/massage
- ○ laughter
- ○ time to myself
- ○ visualized my future
- ○ quality sleep

high quality nourishment

water/hydrating liquids: _____

whole grains: _____

vegetables: _____

fruits: _____

healthy fats: _____

protein: _____

supplements: _____

how i felt today

mood: _____ digestion: _____

energy: _____ cravings: _____

today i appreciate myself for: _____

_____

choices that did not serve me or support me: _____

_____

today i added in or crowded out: _____

_____

loving thought before bed: _____

_____

morning intentions

date: _____

morning thoughts, feelings & intuitions: _____
_____
_____
_____

i am grateful for: _____
_____
_____
_____

goals for today:

○ _____
○ _____
○ _____

action steps for each goal:

○ _____ ○ _____ ○ _____
○ _____ ○ _____ ○ _____
○ _____ ○ _____ ○ _____

fun, relaxation & adventure for today:

○ _____
○ _____
○ _____

evening reflections

○ morning intentions
○ home-cooked food (__x)
○ mindful eating
○ reduced one food
○ tongue scraper
○ hot towel scrub

○ hot water bottle
○ conscious breathing
○ fresh air
○ physical activity
○ prayer/meditation
○ meaningful connections

○ loving work
○ touch/massage
○ laughter
○ time to myself
○ visualized my future
○ quality sleep

high quality nourishment

water/hydrating liquids: _____

whole grains: _____

vegetables: _____

fruits: _____

healthy fats: _____

protein: _____

supplements: _____

how i felt today

mood: _____ digestion: _____

energy: _____ cravings: _____

today i appreciate myself for: _____

_____

choices that did not serve me or support me: _____

_____

today i added in or crowded out: _____

_____

loving thought before bed: _____

_____

morning intentions

date: _____

morning thoughts, feelings & intuitions: _____

_____

_____

_____

i am grateful for: _____

_____

_____

_____

goals for today:

○ _____

○ _____

○ _____

action steps for each goal:

○ _____ ○ _____ ○ _____

○ _____ ○ _____ ○ _____

○ _____ ○ _____ ○ _____

fun, relaxation & adventure for today:

○ _____

○ _____

○ _____

evening reflections

○ morning intentions
○ home-cooked food (__x)
○ mindful eating
○ reduced one food
○ tongue scraper
○ hot towel scrub

○ hot water bottle
○ conscious breathing
○ fresh air
○ physical activity
○ prayer/meditation
○ meaningful connections

○ loving work
○ touch/massage
○ laughter
○ time to myself
○ visualized my future
○ quality sleep

high quality nourishment

water/hydrating liquids: _____

whole grains: _____

vegetables: _____

fruits: _____

healthy fats: _____

protein: _____

supplements: _____

how i felt today

mood: _____ digestion: _____

energy: _____ cravings: _____

today i appreciate myself for: _____

_____

choices that did not serve me or support me: _____

_____

today i added in or crowded out: _____

_____

loving thought before bed: _____

_____

morning intentions

date: _____

morning thoughts, feelings & intuitions: _____

_____

_____

_____

i am grateful for: _____

_____

_____

_____

goals for today:

○ _____

○ _____

○ _____

action steps for each goal:

○ _____ ○ _____ ○ _____

○ _____ ○ _____ ○ _____

○ _____ ○ _____ ○ _____

fun, relaxation & adventure for today:

○ _____

○ _____

○ _____

evening reflections

- ○ morning intentions
- ○ home-cooked food (__x)
- ○ mindful eating
- ○ reduced one food
- ○ tongue scraper
- ○ hot towel scrub

- ○ hot water bottle
- ○ conscious breathing
- ○ fresh air
- ○ physical activity
- ○ prayer/meditation
- ○ meaningful connections

- ○ loving work
- ○ touch/massage
- ○ laughter
- ○ time to myself
- ○ visualized my future
- ○ quality sleep

high quality nourishment

water/hydrating liquids: _____

whole grains: _____

vegetables: _____

fruits: _____

healthy fats: _____

protein: _____

supplements: _____

how i felt today

mood: _____ digestion: _____

energy: _____ cravings: _____

today i appreciate myself for: _____

_____

choices that did not serve me or support me: _____

_____

today i added in or crowded out: _____

_____

loving thought before bed: _____

_____

morning intentions

date: _____

morning thoughts, feelings & intuitions: _____

_____

_____

_____

i am grateful for: _____

_____

_____

_____

goals for today:

◯ _____

◯ _____

◯ _____

action steps for each goal:

◯ _____ ◯ _____ ◯ _____

◯ _____ ◯ _____ ◯ _____

◯ _____ ◯ _____ ◯ _____

fun, relaxation & adventure for today:

◯ _____

◯ _____

◯ _____

evening reflections

○ morning intentions
○ home-cooked food (__x)
○ mindful eating
○ reduced one food
○ tongue scraper
○ hot towel scrub

○ hot water bottle
○ conscious breathing
○ fresh air
○ physical activity
○ prayer/meditation
○ meaningful connections

○ loving work
○ touch/massage
○ laughter
○ time to myself
○ visualized my future
○ quality sleep

high quality nourishment

water/hydrating liquids: _____

whole grains: _____

vegetables: _____

fruits: _____

healthy fats: _____

protein: _____

supplements: _____

how i felt today

mood: _____ digestion: _____

energy: _____ cravings: _____

today i appreciate myself for: _____

_____

choices that did not serve me or support me: _____

_____

today i added in or crowded out: _____

_____

loving thought before bed: _____

_____

weekly check-in

dates: _____

what's new & good?

energy & vitality: _____
_____

chewing & digestion: _____
_____

cravings & addictions: _____
_____

hair & skin: _____
_____

mouth, teeth & tongue: _____
_____

body shape & weight: _____
_____

posture & breathing: _____
_____

mood & emotions: _____
_____

relating to others: _____
_____

about the week

most nourishing food: _____
_____

best primary food: _____
_____

special person i appreciate: _____
_____

biggest challenge: _____
_____

main health concern: _____
_____

greatest accomplishment: _____
_____

most fun i had: _____
_____

i got clear that i really want to: _____
_____

other thoughts: _____
_____

next week I plan to: _____
_____

guided exercise

if money didn't matter

If you decided right now that you had enough money, and that you would always have enough, what would you do with your life?

I would work as a personal chef (for people who are sick as well as others) at an excellent hourly rate + continue to make excellent income -

I'd make my own hours - Work fewer hours + make more $.

Because I loved it, it wouldn't feel like work -

I'd travel more -

Have more time for self - care + to model health) to my clients -

The human body is unlimited in potential,
it is just a matter of knowing how to access it.

John Douillard, PhD

morning intentions

date: _____

morning thoughts, feelings & intuitions: _____

_____

_____

_____

i am grateful for: _____

_____

_____

_____

goals for today:

○ _____

○ _____

○ _____

action steps for each goal:

○ _____ ○ _____ ○ _____

○ _____ ○ _____ ○ _____

○ _____ ○ _____ ○ _____

fun, relaxation & adventure for today:

○ _____

○ _____

○ _____

e v e n i n g   r e f l e c t i o n s

○ morning intentions
○ home-cooked food (__x)
○ mindful eating
○ reduced one food
○ tongue scraper
○ hot towel scrub

○ hot water bottle
○ conscious breathing
○ fresh air
○ physical activity
○ prayer/meditation
○ meaningful connections

○ loving work
○ touch/massage
○ laughter
○ time to myself
○ visualized my future
○ quality sleep

high quality nourishment

water/hydrating liquids: _____

whole grains: _____

vegetables: _____

fruits: _____

healthy fats: _____

protein: _____

supplements: _____

how i felt today

mood: _____   digestion: _____

energy: _____   cravings: _____

today i appreciate myself for: _____

_____

choices that did not serve me or support me: _____

_____

today i added in or crowded out: _____

_____

loving thought before bed: _____

_____

morning intentions

date: _____

morning thoughts, feelings & intuitions: _____

_____

_____

_____

i am grateful for: _____

_____

_____

_____

goals for today:

◯ _____

◯ _____

◯ _____

action steps for each goal:

◯ _____ ◯ _____ ◯ _____

◯ _____ ◯ _____ ◯ _____

◯ _____ ◯ _____ ◯ _____

fun, relaxation & adventure for today:

◯ _____

◯ _____

◯ _____

evening reflections

- ◯ morning intentions
- ◯ home-cooked food (__x)
- ◯ mindful eating
- ◯ reduced one food
- ◯ tongue scraper
- ◯ hot towel scrub

- ◯ hot water bottle
- ◯ conscious breathing
- ◯ fresh air
- ◯ physical activity
- ◯ prayer/meditation
- ◯ meaningful connections

- ◯ loving work
- ◯ touch/massage
- ◯ laughter
- ◯ time to myself
- ◯ visualized my future
- ◯ quality sleep

high quality nourishment

water/hydrating liquids: _____

whole grains: _____

vegetables: _____

fruits: _____

healthy fats: _____

protein: _____

supplements: _____

how i felt today

mood: _____ digestion: _____

energy: _____ cravings: _____

today i appreciate myself for: _____

_____

choices that did not serve me or support me: _____

_____

today i added in or crowded out: _____

_____

loving thought before bed: _____

_____

morning intentions

date: _____

morning thoughts, feelings & intuitions: _____

_____

_____

_____

i am grateful for: _____

_____

_____

_____

goals for today:

○ _____

○ _____

○ _____

action steps for each goal:

○ _____ ○ _____ ○ _____

○ _____ ○ _____ ○ _____

○ _____ ○ _____ ○ _____

fun, relaxation & adventure for today:

○ _____

○ _____

○ _____

evening reflections

○ morning intentions
○ home-cooked food (__x)
○ mindful eating
○ reduced one food
○ tongue scraper
○ hot towel scrub

○ hot water bottle
○ conscious breathing
○ fresh air
○ physical activity
○ prayer/meditation
○ meaningful connections

○ loving work
○ touch/massage
○ laughter
○ time to myself
○ visualized my future
○ quality sleep

high quality nourishment

water/hydrating liquids: _____

whole grains: _____

vegetables: _____

fruits: _____

healthy fats: _____

protein: _____

supplements: _____

how i felt today

mood: _____   digestion: _____

energy: _____   cravings: _____

today i appreciate myself for: _____

_____

choices that did not serve me or support me: _____

_____

today i added in or crowded out: _____

_____

loving thought before bed: _____

_____

morning intentions

date: _____

morning thoughts, feelings & intuitions: _____

_____

_____

_____

i am grateful for: _____

_____

_____

_____

goals for today:

○ _____

○ _____

○ _____

action steps for each goal:

○ _____ ○ _____ ○ _____

○ _____ ○ _____ ○ _____

○ _____ ○ _____ ○ _____

fun, relaxation & adventure for today:

○ _____

○ _____

○ _____

evening reflections

- ◯ morning intentions
- ◯ home-cooked food (__x)
- ◯ mindful eating
- ◯ reduced one food
- ◯ tongue scraper
- ◯ hot towel scrub

- ◯ hot water bottle
- ◯ conscious breathing
- ◯ fresh air
- ◯ physical activity
- ◯ prayer/meditation
- ◯ meaningful connections

- ◯ loving work
- ◯ touch/massage
- ◯ laughter
- ◯ time to myself
- ◯ visualized my future
- ◯ quality sleep

high quality nourishment

water/hydrating liquids: _____

whole grains: _____

vegetables: _____

fruits: _____

healthy fats: _____

protein: _____

supplements: _____

how i felt today

mood: _____   digestion: _____

energy: _____   cravings: _____

today i appreciate myself for: _____

_____

choices that did not serve me or support me: _____

_____

today i added in or crowded out: _____

_____

loving thought before bed: _____

_____

morning intentions

date: _____

morning thoughts, feelings & intuitions: _____
_____
_____
_____

i am grateful for: _____
_____
_____
_____

goals for today:

◯ _____
◯ _____
◯ _____

action steps for each goal:

◯ _____ ◯ _____ ◯ _____
◯ _____ ◯ _____ ◯ _____
◯ _____ ◯ _____ ◯ _____

fun, relaxation & adventure for today:

◯ _____
◯ _____
◯ _____

evening reflections

○ morning intentions   ○ hot water bottle   ○ loving work
○ home-cooked food (__x)   ○ conscious breathing   ○ touch/massage
○ mindful eating   ○ fresh air   ○ laughter
○ reduced one food   ○ physical activity   ○ time to myself
○ tongue scraper   ○ prayer/meditation   ○ visualized my future
○ hot towel scrub   ○ meaningful connections   ○ quality sleep

high quality nourishment

water/hydrating liquids: _____

whole grains: _____

vegetables: _____

fruits: _____

healthy fats: _____

protein: _____

supplements: _____

how i felt today

mood: _____   digestion: _____

energy: _____   cravings: _____

today i appreciate myself for: _____

_____

choices that did not serve me or support me: _____

_____

today i added in or crowded out: _____

_____

loving thought before bed: _____

_____

morning intentions

date: _____

morning thoughts, feelings & intuitions: _____

_____

_____

_____

i am grateful for: _____

_____

_____

_____

goals for today:

○ _____

○ _____

○ _____

action steps for each goal:

○ _____ ○ _____ ○ _____

○ _____ ○ _____ ○ _____

○ _____ ○ _____ ○ _____

fun, relaxation & adventure for today:

○ _____

○ _____

○ _____

evening reflections

- ○ morning intentions
- ○ home-cooked food (__x)
- ○ mindful eating
- ○ reduced one food
- ○ tongue scraper
- ○ hot towel scrub

- ○ hot water bottle
- ○ conscious breathing
- ○ fresh air
- ○ physical activity
- ○ prayer/meditation
- ○ meaningful connections

- ○ loving work
- ○ touch/massage
- ○ laughter
- ○ time to myself
- ○ visualized my future
- ○ quality sleep

high quality nourishment

water/hydrating liquids: _____

whole grains: _____

vegetables: _____

fruits: _____

healthy fats: _____

protein: _____

supplements: _____

how i felt today

mood: _____ digestion: _____

energy: _____ cravings: _____

today i appreciate myself for: _____

_____

choices that did not serve me or support me: _____

_____

today i added in or crowded out: _____

_____

loving thought before bed: _____

_____

morning intentions

date: _____

morning thoughts, feelings & intuitions: _____

_____

_____

_____

i am grateful for: _____

_____

_____

_____

goals for today:

○ _____

○ _____

○ _____

action steps for each goal:

○ _____ ○ _____ ○ _____

○ _____ ○ _____ ○ _____

○ _____ ○ _____ ○ _____

fun, relaxation & adventure for today:

○ _____

○ _____

○ _____

e v e n i n g   r e f l e c t i o n s

- ◯ morning intentions
- ◯ home-cooked food (__x)
- ◯ mindful eating
- ◯ reduced one food
- ◯ tongue scraper
- ◯ hot towel scrub

- ◯ hot water bottle
- ◯ conscious breathing
- ◯ fresh air
- ◯ physical activity
- ◯ prayer/meditation
- ◯ meaningful connections

- ◯ loving work
- ◯ touch/massage
- ◯ laughter
- ◯ time to myself
- ◯ visualized my future
- ◯ quality sleep

high quality nourishment

water/hydrating liquids: _____

whole grains: _____

vegetables: _____

fruits: _____

healthy fats: _____

protein: _____

supplements: _____

how i felt today

mood: _____ digestion: _____

energy: _____ cravings: _____

today i appreciate myself for: _____

_____

choices that did not serve me or support me: _____

_____

today i added in or crowded out: _____

_____

loving thought before bed: _____

_____

weekly check-in

dates: _____

what's new & good?

energy & vitality: _____
_____

chewing & digestion: _____
_____

cravings & addictions: _____
_____

hair & skin: _____
_____

mouth, teeth & tongue: _____
_____

body shape & weight: _____
_____

posture & breathing: _____
_____

mood & emotions: _____
_____

relating to others: _____
_____

about the week

most nourishing food: _____

_____

best primary food: _____

_____

special person i appreciate: _____

_____

biggest challenge: _____

_____

main health concern: _____

_____

greatest accomplishment: _____

_____

most fun i had: _____

_____

i got clear that i really want to: _____

_____

other thoughts: _____

_____

next week I plan to: _____

_____

guided exercise

love letter

Ask someone in your life to write you a letter about everything
they love about you. Have them write it in these pages,
or if they give it to you separately, paste it into the journal.

When something archetypal possesses you, you're actually owned by that energy. It's not something you keep pumping up. It keeps flowing through you and you feel alive and energized, and more ideas come and more structure comes, and after awhile you have a vision.

Harville Hendrix, PhD

morning intentions

date: _____

morning thoughts, feelings & intuitions: _____

_____

_____

_____

i am grateful for: _____

_____

_____

_____

goals for today:

○ _____

○ _____

○ _____

action steps for each goal:

○ _____ ○ _____ ○ _____

○ _____ ○ _____ ○ _____

○ _____ ○ _____ ○ _____

fun, relaxation & adventure for today:

○ _____

○ _____

○ _____

evening reflections

- ○ morning intentions
- ○ home-cooked food (__x)
- ○ mindful eating
- ○ reduced one food
- ○ tongue scraper
- ○ hot towel scrub

- ○ hot water bottle
- ○ conscious breathing
- ○ fresh air
- ○ physical activity
- ○ prayer/meditation
- ○ meaningful connections

- ○ loving work
- ○ touch/massage
- ○ laughter
- ○ time to myself
- ○ visualized my future
- ○ quality sleep

high quality nourishment

water/hydrating liquids: _____

whole grains: _____

vegetables: _____

fruits: _____

healthy fats: _____

protein: _____

supplements: _____

how i felt today

mood: _____ digestion: _____

energy: _____ cravings: _____

today i appreciate myself for: _____

_____

choices that did not serve me or support me: _____

_____

today i added in or crowded out: _____

_____

loving thought before bed: _____

_____

morning intentions

date: _____

morning thoughts, feelings & intuitions: _____

_____

_____

_____

i am grateful for: _____

_____

_____

_____

goals for today:

◯ _____

◯ _____

◯ _____

action steps for each goal:

◯ _____   ◯ _____   ◯ _____

◯ _____   ◯ _____   ◯ _____

◯ _____   ◯ _____   ◯ _____

fun, relaxation & adventure for today:

◯ _____

◯ _____

◯ _____

evening reflections

- ○ morning intentions
- ○ home-cooked food (__x)
- ○ mindful eating
- ○ reduced one food
- ○ tongue scraper
- ○ hot towel scrub

- ○ hot water bottle
- ○ conscious breathing
- ○ fresh air
- ○ physical activity
- ○ prayer/meditation
- ○ meaningful connections

- ○ loving work
- ○ touch/massage
- ○ laughter
- ○ time to myself
- ○ visualized my future
- ○ quality sleep

high quality nourishment

water/hydrating liquids: _____

whole grains: _____

vegetables: _____

fruits: _____

healthy fats: _____

protein: _____

supplements: _____

how i felt today

mood: _____   digestion: _____

energy: _____   cravings: _____

today i appreciate myself for: _____

_____

choices that did not serve me or support me: _____

_____

today i added in or crowded out: _____

_____

loving thought before bed: _____

_____

morning intentions

date: _____

morning thoughts, feelings & intuitions: _____

_____

_____

_____

i am grateful for: _____

_____

_____

_____

goals for today:

O _____

O _____

O _____

action steps for each goal:

O _____ O _____ O _____

O _____ O _____ O _____

O _____ O _____ O _____

fun, relaxation & adventure for today:

O _____

O _____

O _____

evening reflections

- ○ morning intentions
- ○ home-cooked food (__x)
- ○ mindful eating
- ○ reduced one food
- ○ tongue scraper
- ○ hot towel scrub

- ○ hot water bottle
- ○ conscious breathing
- ○ fresh air
- ○ physical activity
- ○ prayer/meditation
- ○ meaningful connections

- ○ loving work
- ○ touch/massage
- ○ laughter
- ○ time to myself
- ○ visualized my future
- ○ quality sleep

high quality nourishment

water/hydrating liquids: _____

whole grains: _____

vegetables: _____

fruits: _____

healthy fats: _____

protein: _____

supplements: _____

how i felt today

mood: _____ digestion: _____

energy: _____ cravings: _____

today i appreciate myself for: _____

_____

choices that did not serve me or support me: _____

_____

today i added in or crowded out: _____

_____

loving thought before bed: _____

_____

morning intentions

date: _____

morning thoughts, feelings & intuitions: _____

_____

_____

_____

i am grateful for: _____

_____

_____

_____

goals for today:

○ _____

○ _____

○ _____

action steps for each goal:

○ _____ ○ _____ ○ _____

○ _____ ○ _____ ○ _____

○ _____ ○ _____ ○ _____

fun, relaxation & adventure for today:

○ _____

○ _____

○ _____

evening reflections

○ morning intentions
○ home-cooked food (__x)
○ mindful eating
○ reduced one food
○ tongue scraper
○ hot towel scrub

○ hot water bottle
○ conscious breathing
○ fresh air
○ physical activity
○ prayer/meditation
○ meaningful connections

○ loving work
○ touch/massage
○ laughter
○ time to myself
○ visualized my future
○ quality sleep

high quality nourishment

water/hydrating liquids: _____

whole grains: _____

vegetables: _____

fruits: _____

healthy fats: _____

protein: _____

supplements: _____

how i felt today

mood: _____ digestion: _____

energy: _____ cravings: _____

today i appreciate myself for: _____
_____

choices that did not serve me or support me: _____
_____

today i added in or crowded out: _____
_____

loving thought before bed: _____
_____

morning intentions

date: _____

morning thoughts, feelings & intuitions: _____
_____
_____
_____

i am grateful for: _____
_____
_____
_____

goals for today:

○ _____
○ _____
○ _____

action steps for each goal:

○ _____ ○ _____ ○ _____
○ _____ ○ _____ ○ _____
○ _____ ○ _____ ○ _____

fun, relaxation & adventure for today:

○ _____
○ _____
○ _____

evening reflections

○ morning intentions
○ home-cooked food (__x)
○ mindful eating
○ reduced one food
○ tongue scraper
○ hot towel scrub

○ hot water bottle
○ conscious breathing
○ fresh air
○ physical activity
○ prayer/meditation
○ meaningful connections

○ loving work
○ touch/massage
○ laughter
○ time to myself
○ visualized my future
○ quality sleep

high quality nourishment

water/hydrating liquids: _____

whole grains: _____

vegetables: _____

fruits: _____

healthy fats: _____

protein: _____

supplements: _____

how i felt today

mood: _____   digestion: _____

energy: _____   cravings: _____

today i appreciate myself for: _____

_____

choices that did not serve me or support me: _____

_____

today i added in or crowded out: _____

_____

loving thought before bed: _____

_____

morning intentions

date: _____

morning thoughts, feelings & intuitions: _____

_____

_____

_____

i am grateful for: _____

_____

_____

_____

goals for today:

○ _____

○ _____

○ _____

action steps for each goal:

○ _____ ○ _____ ○ _____

○ _____ ○ _____ ○ _____

○ _____ ○ _____ ○ _____

fun, relaxation & adventure for today:

○ _____

○ _____

○ _____

evening reflections

○ morning intentions
○ home-cooked food (__x)
○ mindful eating
○ reduced one food
○ tongue scraper
○ hot towel scrub

○ hot water bottle
○ conscious breathing
○ fresh air
○ physical activity
○ prayer/meditation
○ meaningful connections

○ loving work
○ touch/massage
○ laughter
○ time to myself
○ visualized my future
○ quality sleep

high quality nourishment

water/hydrating liquids: _____

whole grains: _____

vegetables: _____

fruits: _____

healthy fats: _____

protein: _____

supplements: _____

how i felt today

mood: _____ digestion: _____

energy: _____ cravings: _____

today i appreciate myself for: _____

_____

choices that did not serve me or support me: _____

_____

today i added in or crowded out: _____

_____

loving thought before bed: _____

_____

morning intentions

date: _____

morning thoughts, feelings & intuitions: _____

_____

_____

_____

i am grateful for: _____

_____

_____

_____

goals for today:

○ _____

○ _____

○ _____

action steps for each goal:

○ _____ ○ _____ ○ _____

○ _____ ○ _____ ○ _____

○ _____ ○ _____ ○ _____

fun, relaxation & adventure for today:

○ _____

○ _____

○ _____

evening reflections

- ○ morning intentions
- ○ home-cooked food (__x)
- ○ mindful eating
- ○ reduced one food
- ○ tongue scraper
- ○ hot towel scrub

- ○ hot water bottle
- ○ conscious breathing
- ○ fresh air
- ○ physical activity
- ○ prayer/meditation
- ○ meaningful connections

- ○ loving work
- ○ touch/massage
- ○ laughter
- ○ time to myself
- ○ visualized my future
- ○ quality sleep

high quality nourishment

water/hydrating liquids: _____

whole grains: _____

vegetables: _____

fruits: _____

healthy fats: _____

protein: _____

supplements: _____

how i felt today

mood: _____ digestion: _____

energy: _____ cravings: _____

today i appreciate myself for: _____

_____

choices that did not serve me or support me: _____

_____

today i added in or crowded out: _____

_____

loving thought before bed: _____

_____

weekly check-in

dates: _____

what's new & good?

energy & vitality: _____
_____

chewing & digestion: _____
_____

cravings & addictions: _____
_____

hair & skin: _____
_____

mouth, teeth & tongue: _____
_____

body shape & weight: _____
_____

posture & breathing: _____
_____

mood & emotions: _____
_____

relating to others: _____
_____

about the week

most nourishing food: _____

_____

best primary food: _____

_____

special person i appreciate: _____

_____

biggest challenge: _____

_____

main health concern: _____

_____

greatest accomplishment: _____

_____

most fun i had: _____

_____

i got clear that i really want to: _____

_____

other thoughts: _____

_____

next week I plan to: _____

_____

guided exercise

creating my future

Picture yourself 10 years from now.

What are you doing?

Where are you living?

Who is in your life?

What is important to you?

What have you achieved and experienced?

Show up, not just for meals, but for your life.

Geneen Roth

morning intentions

date: _____

morning thoughts, feelings & intuitions: _____

_____

_____

_____

i am grateful for: _____

_____

_____

_____

goals for today:

○ _____

○ _____

○ _____

action steps for each goal:

○ _____ ○ _____ ○ _____

○ _____ ○ _____ ○ _____

○ _____ ○ _____ ○ _____

fun, relaxation & adventure for today:

○ _____

○ _____

○ _____

evening reflections

○ morning intentions
○ home-cooked food (__x)
○ mindful eating
○ reduced one food
○ tongue scraper
○ hot towel scrub

○ hot water bottle
○ conscious breathing
○ fresh air
○ physical activity
○ prayer/meditation
○ meaningful connections

○ loving work
○ touch/massage
○ laughter
○ time to myself
○ visualized my future
○ quality sleep

high quality nourishment

water/hydrating liquids: _____

whole grains: _____

vegetables: _____

fruits: _____

healthy fats: _____

protein: _____

supplements: _____

how i felt today

mood: _____ digestion: _____

energy: _____ cravings: _____

today i appreciate myself for: _____

_____

choices that did not serve me or support me: _____

_____

today i added in or crowded out: _____

_____

loving thought before bed: _____

_____

morning intentions

date: _____

morning thoughts, feelings & intuitions: _____

_____

_____

_____

i am grateful for: _____

_____

_____

_____

goals for today:

○ _____

○ _____

○ _____

action steps for each goal:

○ _____ ○ _____ ○ _____

○ _____ ○ _____ ○ _____

○ _____ ○ _____ ○ _____

fun, relaxation & adventure for today:

○ _____

○ _____

○ _____

evening reflections

- ○ morning intentions
- ○ home-cooked food (__x)
- ○ mindful eating
- ○ reduced one food
- ○ tongue scraper
- ○ hot towel scrub

- ○ hot water bottle
- ○ conscious breathing
- ○ fresh air
- ○ physical activity
- ○ prayer/meditation
- ○ meaningful connections

- ○ loving work
- ○ touch/massage
- ○ laughter
- ○ time to myself
- ○ visualized my future
- ○ quality sleep

high quality nourishment

water/hydrating liquids: _____

whole grains: _____

vegetables: _____

fruits: _____

healthy fats: _____

protein: _____

supplements: _____

how i felt today

mood: _____ digestion: _____

energy: _____ cravings: _____

today i appreciate myself for: _____

_____

choices that did not serve me or support me: _____

_____

today i added in or crowded out: _____

_____

loving thought before bed: _____

_____

morning intentions

date: _____

morning thoughts, feelings & intuitions: _____

_____

_____

_____

i am grateful for: _____

_____

_____

_____

goals for today:

○ _____

○ _____

○ _____

action steps for each goal:

○ _____ ○ _____ ○ _____

○ _____ ○ _____ ○ _____

○ _____ ○ _____ ○ _____

fun, relaxation & adventure for today:

○ _____

○ _____

○ _____

evening reflections

○ morning intentions
○ home-cooked food (__x)
○ mindful eating
○ reduced one food
○ tongue scraper
○ hot towel scrub

○ hot water bottle
○ conscious breathing
○ fresh air
○ physical activity
○ prayer/meditation
○ meaningful connections

○ loving work
○ touch/massage
○ laughter
○ time to myself
○ visualized my future
○ quality sleep

high quality nourishment

water/hydrating liquids: _____

whole grains: _____

vegetables: _____

fruits: _____

healthy fats: _____

protein: _____

supplements: _____

how i felt today

mood: _____ digestion: _____

energy: _____ cravings: _____

today i appreciate myself for: _____

_____

choices that did not serve me or support me: _____

_____

today i added in or crowded out: _____

_____

loving thought before bed: _____

_____

morning intentions

date: _____

morning thoughts, feelings & intuitions: _____

_____

_____

_____

i am grateful for: _____

_____

_____

_____

goals for today:

○ _____

○ _____

○ _____

action steps for each goal:

○ _____ ○ _____ ○ _____

○ _____ ○ _____ ○ _____

○ _____ ○ _____ ○ _____

fun, relaxation & adventure for today:

○ _____

○ _____

○ _____

evening reflections

○ morning intentions   ○ hot water bottle   ○ loving work
○ home-cooked food (__x) ○ conscious breathing ○ touch/massage
○ mindful eating   ○ fresh air   ○ laughter
○ reduced one food   ○ physical activity   ○ time to myself
○ tongue scraper   ○ prayer/meditation   ○ visualized my future
○ hot towel scrub   ○ meaningful connections ○ quality sleep

high quality nourishment

water/hydrating liquids: _____

whole grains: _____

vegetables: _____

fruits: _____

healthy fats: _____

protein: _____

supplements: _____

how i felt today

mood: _____ digestion: _____

energy: _____ cravings: _____

today i appreciate myself for: _____

_____

choices that did not serve me or support me: _____

_____

today i added in or crowded out: _____

_____

loving thought before bed: _____

_____

morning intentions

date: _____

morning thoughts, feelings & intuitions: _____

_____

_____

_____

i am grateful for: _____

_____

_____

_____

goals for today:

○ _____

○ _____

○ _____

action steps for each goal:

○ _____ ○ _____ ○ _____

○ _____ ○ _____ ○ _____

○ _____ ○ _____ ○ _____

fun, relaxation & adventure for today:

○ _____

○ _____

○ _____

evening reflections

- ○ morning intentions
- ○ home-cooked food (__x)
- ○ mindful eating
- ○ reduced one food
- ○ tongue scraper
- ○ hot towel scrub

- ○ hot water bottle
- ○ conscious breathing
- ○ fresh air
- ○ physical activity
- ○ prayer/meditation
- ○ meaningful connections

- ○ loving work
- ○ touch/massage
- ○ laughter
- ○ time to myself
- ○ visualized my future
- ○ quality sleep

high quality nourishment

water/hydrating liquids: _____

whole grains: _____

vegetables: _____

fruits: _____

healthy fats: _____

protein: _____

supplements: _____

how i felt today

mood: _____ digestion: _____

energy: _____ cravings: _____

today i appreciate myself for: _____

_____

choices that did not serve me or support me: _____

_____

today i added in or crowded out: _____

_____

loving thought before bed: _____

_____

morning intentions

date: _____

morning thoughts, feelings & intuitions: _____

_____

_____

_____

i am grateful for: _____

_____

_____

_____

goals for today:

◯ _____

◯ _____

◯ _____

action steps for each goal:

◯ _____ ◯ _____ ◯ _____

◯ _____ ◯ _____ ◯ _____

◯ _____ ◯ _____ ◯ _____

fun, relaxation & adventure for today:

◯ _____

◯ _____

◯ _____

evening reflections

○ morning intentions
○ home-cooked food (__x)
○ mindful eating
○ reduced one food
○ tongue scraper
○ hot towel scrub

○ hot water bottle
○ conscious breathing
○ fresh air
○ physical activity
○ prayer/meditation
○ meaningful connections

○ loving work
○ touch/massage
○ laughter
○ time to myself
○ visualized my future
○ quality sleep

high quality nourishment

water/hydrating liquids: _____

whole grains: _____

vegetables: _____

fruits: _____

healthy fats: _____

protein: _____

supplements: _____

how i felt today

mood: _____ digestion: _____

energy: _____ cravings: _____

today i appreciate myself for: _____

_____

choices that did not serve me or support me: _____

_____

today i added in or crowded out: _____

_____

loving thought before bed: _____

_____

morning intentions

date: _____

morning thoughts, feelings & intuitions: _____
_____
_____
_____

i am grateful for: _____
_____
_____
_____

goals for today:

O _____
O _____
O _____

action steps for each goal:

O _____ O _____ O _____
O _____ O _____ O _____
O _____ O _____ O _____

fun, relaxation & adventure for today:

O _____
O _____
O _____

evening reflections

- ○ morning intentions
- ○ home-cooked food (__x)
- ○ mindful eating
- ○ reduced one food
- ○ tongue scraper
- ○ hot towel scrub

- ○ hot water bottle
- ○ conscious breathing
- ○ fresh air
- ○ physical activity
- ○ prayer/meditation
- ○ meaningful connections

- ○ loving work
- ○ touch/massage
- ○ laughter
- ○ time to myself
- ○ visualized my future
- ○ quality sleep

high quality nourishment

water/hydrating liquids: _____

whole grains: _____

vegetables: _____

fruits: _____

healthy fats: _____

protein: _____

supplements: _____

how i felt today

mood: _____ digestion: _____

energy: _____ cravings: _____

today i appreciate myself for: _____

_____

choices that did not serve me or support me: _____

_____

today i added in or crowded out: _____

_____

loving thought before bed: _____

_____

month one progress

dates: _____

what's changed this month?

food & cooking: _____
_____
_____

self-care: _____
_____
_____

physical health: _____
_____
_____

main health concern: _____
_____
_____

habits, cravings & addictions: _____
_____
_____

moods, thoughts & feelings: _____
_____
_____

primary food progress

career: _____

_____

relationships: _____

_____

physical activity: _____

_____

spirituality: _____

_____

creativity: _____

_____

fun, relaxation & adventure: _____

_____

other accomplishments: _____

_____

_____

_____

_____

_____

Eat less, move more, eat lots of fruits and vegetables, go easy on junk foods.

Marion Nestle, PhD, MPH

Each person's ideal diet is discovered
through a combination of study,
observation and intuition.

Sally Fallon, MA

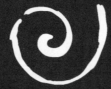

month two

circle of life

This exercise will help you discover which primary foods need attention in order for you to create more balance in your life. The circle has twelve sections. Place a dot on the line for each section to designate how satisfied you are with that aspect of your life. A dot placed towards the center of the circle indicates dissatisfaction, while a dot placed towards the periphery indicates ultimate happiness. When you have placed a dot on each line, connect the dots to see your Circle of Life. Now you have a clear visual of any areas that may need your attention. You will complete this exercise again next month to see if your circle has become more balanced.

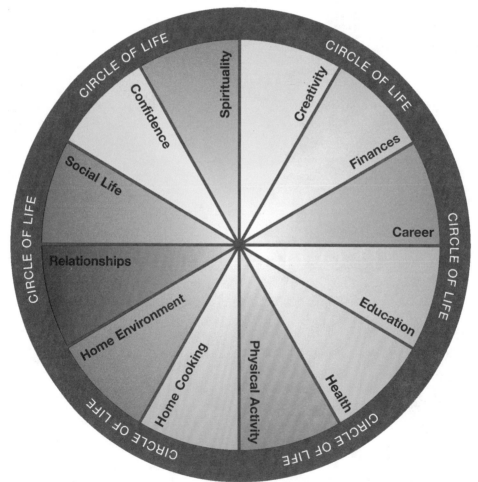

wish list

Now that you have identified areas of your life that are out of balance or unsatisfying, what would it take to bring them into balance? What experiences, items, relationships or feelings would make those parts of your life juicy and exciting? This exercise will help you get in touch with your desires. In the table below, begin listing simple and obvious wishes. Bigger, more exciting desires will come as you write.

Keep these desires in mind when setting your morning intentions. Whenever you fulfill a desire, put an X in the "done" column. In the "gratitude" column, thank anyone who may have helped. You might be thanking yourself. Notice how, as you take better care of yourself, your desires naturally come true, and your life becomes more fulfilling.

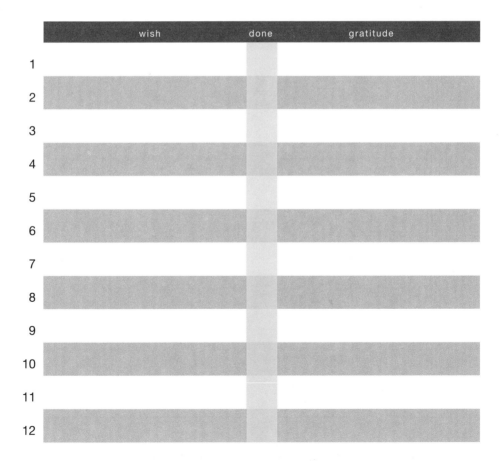

	wish	done	gratitude
1			
2			
3			
4			
5			
6			
7			
8			
9			
10			
11			
12			

morning intentions

date: _____

morning thoughts, feelings & intuitions: _____

_____

_____

_____

i am grateful for: _____

_____

_____

_____

goals for today:

○ _____

○ _____

○ _____

action steps for each goal:

○ _____ ○ _____ ○ _____

○ _____ ○ _____ ○ _____

○ _____ ○ _____ ○ _____

fun, relaxation & adventure for today:

○ _____

○ _____

○ _____

evening reflections

○ morning intentions
○ home-cooked food (__x)
○ mindful eating
○ reduced one food
○ tongue scraper
○ hot towel scrub

○ hot water bottle
○ conscious breathing
○ fresh air
○ physical activity
○ prayer/meditation
○ meaningful connections

○ loving work
○ touch/massage
○ laughter
○ time to myself
○ visualized my future
○ quality sleep

high quality nourishment

water/hydrating liquids: _____

whole grains: _____

vegetables: _____

fruits: _____

healthy fats: _____

protein: _____

supplements: _____

how i felt today

mood: _____ digestion: _____

energy: _____ cravings: _____

today i appreciate myself for: _____

_____

choices that did not serve me or support me: _____

_____

today i added in or crowded out: _____

_____

loving thought before bed: _____

_____

morning intentions

date: _____

morning thoughts, feelings & intuitions: _____

_____

_____

_____

i am grateful for: _____

_____

_____

_____

goals for today:

○ _____

○ _____

○ _____

action steps for each goal:

○ _____ ○ _____ ○ _____

○ _____ ○ _____ ○ _____

○ _____ ○ _____ ○ _____

fun, relaxation & adventure for today:

○ _____

○ _____

○ _____

evening reflections

- ○ morning intentions
- ○ home-cooked food (__x)
- ○ mindful eating
- ○ reduced one food
- ○ tongue scraper
- ○ hot towel scrub

- ○ hot water bottle
- ○ conscious breathing
- ○ fresh air
- ○ physical activity
- ○ prayer/meditation
- ○ meaningful connections

- ○ loving work
- ○ touch/massage
- ○ laughter
- ○ time to myself
- ○ visualized my future
- ○ quality sleep

high quality nourishment

water/hydrating liquids: _____

whole grains: _____

vegetables: _____

fruits: _____

healthy fats: _____

protein: _____

supplements: _____

how i felt today

mood: _____ digestion: _____

energy: _____ cravings: _____

today i appreciate myself for: _____

_____

choices that did not serve me or support me: _____

_____

today i added in or crowded out: _____

_____

loving thought before bed: _____

_____

morning intentions

date: _____

morning thoughts, feelings & intuitions: _____

_____

_____

_____

i am grateful for: _____

_____

_____

_____

goals for today:

O _____

O _____

O _____

action steps for each goal:

O _____ O _____ O _____

O _____ O _____ O _____

O _____ O _____ O _____

fun, relaxation & adventure for today:

O _____

O _____

O _____

evening reflections

○ morning intentions
○ home-cooked food (__x)
○ mindful eating
○ reduced one food
○ tongue scraper
○ hot towel scrub

○ hot water bottle
○ conscious breathing
○ fresh air
○ physical activity
○ prayer/meditation
○ meaningful connections

○ loving work
○ touch/massage
○ laughter
○ time to myself
○ visualized my future
○ quality sleep

high quality nourishment

water/hydrating liquids: _____

whole grains: _____

vegetables: _____

fruits: _____

healthy fats: _____

protein: _____

supplements: _____

how i felt today

mood: _____   digestion: _____

energy: _____   cravings: _____

today i appreciate myself for: _____

_____

choices that did not serve me or support me: _____

_____

today i added in or crowded out: _____

_____

loving thought before bed: _____

_____

morning intentions

date: _____

morning thoughts, feelings & intuitions: _____

_____

_____

_____

i am grateful for: _____

_____

_____

_____

goals for today:

○ _____

○ _____

○ _____

action steps for each goal:

○ _____ ○ _____ ○ _____

○ _____ ○ _____ ○ _____

○ _____ ○ _____ ○ _____

fun, relaxation & adventure for today:

○ _____

○ _____

○ _____

evening reflections

- ◯ morning intentions
- ◯ home-cooked food (__x)
- ◯ mindful eating
- ◯ reduced one food
- ◯ tongue scraper
- ◯ hot towel scrub

- ◯ hot water bottle
- ◯ conscious breathing
- ◯ fresh air
- ◯ physical activity
- ◯ prayer/meditation
- ◯ meaningful connections

- ◯ loving work
- ◯ touch/massage
- ◯ laughter
- ◯ time to myself
- ◯ visualized my future
- ◯ quality sleep

high quality nourishment

water/hydrating liquids: _____

whole grains: _____

vegetables: _____

fruits: _____

healthy fats: _____

protein: _____

supplements: _____

how i felt today

mood: _____   digestion: _____

energy: _____   cravings: _____

today i appreciate myself for: _____

_____

choices that did not serve me or support me: _____

_____

today i added in or crowded out: _____

_____

loving thought before bed: _____

_____

morning intentions

date: _____

morning thoughts, feelings & intuitions: _____

_____

_____

_____

i am grateful for: _____

_____

_____

_____

goals for today:

◯ _____

◯ _____

◯ _____

action steps for each goal:

◯ _____ ◯ _____ ◯ _____

◯ _____ ◯ _____ ◯ _____

◯ _____ ◯ _____ ◯ _____

fun, relaxation & adventure for today:

◯ _____

◯ _____

◯ _____

evening reflections

○ morning intentions
○ home-cooked food (__x)
○ mindful eating
○ reduced one food
○ tongue scraper
○ hot towel scrub

○ hot water bottle
○ conscious breathing
○ fresh air
○ physical activity
○ prayer/meditation
○ meaningful connections

○ loving work
○ touch/massage
○ laughter
○ time to myself
○ visualized my future
○ quality sleep

high quality nourishment

water/hydrating liquids: _____

whole grains: _____

vegetables: _____

fruits: _____

healthy fats: _____

protein: _____

supplements: _____

how i felt today

mood: _____   digestion: _____

energy: _____   cravings: _____

today i appreciate myself for: _____

_____

choices that did not serve me or support me: _____

_____

today i added in or crowded out: _____

_____

loving thought before bed: _____

_____

morning intentions

date: _____

morning thoughts, feelings & intuitions: _____

_____

_____

_____

i am grateful for: _____

_____

_____

_____

goals for today:

○ _____

○ _____

○ _____

action steps for each goal:

○ _____ ○ _____ ○ _____

○ _____ ○ _____ ○ _____

○ _____ ○ _____ ○ _____

fun, relaxation & adventure for today:

○ _____

○ _____

○ _____

evening reflections

○ morning intentions   ○ hot water bottle   ○ loving work
○ home-cooked food (__x) ○ conscious breathing ○ touch/massage
○ mindful eating   ○ fresh air   ○ laughter
○ reduced one food   ○ physical activity   ○ time to myself
○ tongue scraper   ○ prayer/meditation   ○ visualized my future
○ hot towel scrub   ○ meaningful connections ○ quality sleep

high quality nourishment

water/hydrating liquids: _____

whole grains: _____

vegetables: _____

fruits: _____

healthy fats: _____

protein: _____

supplements: _____

how i felt today

mood: _____   digestion: _____

energy: _____   cravings: _____

today i appreciate myself for: _____

_____

choices that did not serve me or support me: _____

_____

today i added in or crowded out: _____

_____

loving thought before bed: _____

_____

morning intentions

date: _____

morning thoughts, feelings & intuitions: _____

_____

_____

_____

i am grateful for: _____

_____

_____

_____

goals for today:

○ _____

○ _____

○ _____

action steps for each goal:

○ _____ ○ _____ ○ _____

○ _____ ○ _____ ○ _____

○ _____ ○ _____ ○ _____

fun, relaxation & adventure for today:

○ _____

○ _____

○ _____

evening reflections

○ morning intentions
○ home-cooked food (__x)
○ mindful eating
○ reduced one food
○ tongue scraper
○ hot towel scrub

○ hot water bottle
○ conscious breathing
○ fresh air
○ physical activity
○ prayer/meditation
○ meaningful connections

○ loving work
○ touch/massage
○ laughter
○ time to myself
○ visualized my future
○ quality sleep

high quality nourishment

water/hydrating liquids: _____

whole grains: _____

vegetables: _____

fruits: _____

healthy fats: _____

protein: _____

supplements: _____

how i felt today

mood: _____ digestion: _____

energy: _____ cravings: _____

today i appreciate myself for: _____

_____

choices that did not serve me or support me: _____

_____

today i added in or crowded out: _____

_____

loving thought before bed: _____

_____

weekly check-in

dates: _____

what's new & good?

energy & vitality: _____
_____

chewing & digestion: _____
_____

cravings & addictions: _____
_____

hair & skin: _____
_____

mouth, teeth & tongue: _____
_____

body shape & weight: _____
_____

posture & breathing: _____
_____

mood & emotions: _____
_____

relating to others: _____
_____

about the week

most nourishing food: _____

_____

best primary food: _____

_____

special person i appreciate: _____

_____

biggest challenge: _____

_____

main health concern: _____

_____

greatest accomplishment: _____

_____

most fun i had: _____

_____

i got clear that i really want to: _____

_____

other thoughts: _____

_____

next week I plan to: _____

_____

guided exercise

letting go letter

Who is someone in your life with whom you have an unresolved issue?

Use this space to write them a letter and express
any thoughts or feelings you are still holding on to.

Simply being more aware of imbalance
is the first step to becoming more balanced.

Paul Pitchford, MS

morning intentions

date: _____

morning thoughts, feelings & intuitions: _____

_____

_____

_____

i am grateful for: _____

_____

_____

_____

goals for today:

○ _____

○ _____

○ _____

action steps for each goal:

○ _____ ○ _____ ○ _____

○ _____ ○ _____ ○ _____

○ _____ ○ _____ ○ _____

fun, relaxation & adventure for today:

○ _____

○ _____

○ _____

evening reflections

○ morning intentions
○ home-cooked food (__x)
○ mindful eating
○ reduced one food
○ tongue scraper
○ hot towel scrub

○ hot water bottle
○ conscious breathing
○ fresh air
○ physical activity
○ prayer/meditation
○ meaningful connections

○ loving work
○ touch/massage
○ laughter
○ time to myself
○ visualized my future
○ quality sleep

high quality nourishment

water/hydrating liquids: _____

whole grains: _____

vegetables: _____

fruits: _____

healthy fats: _____

protein: _____

supplements: _____

how i felt today

mood: _____ digestion: _____

energy: _____ cravings: _____

today i appreciate myself for: _____

_____

choices that did not serve me or support me: _____

_____

today i added in or crowded out: _____

_____

loving thought before bed: _____

_____

morning intentions

date: _____

morning thoughts, feelings & intuitions: _____

_____

_____

_____

i am grateful for: _____

_____

_____

_____

goals for today:

O _____

O _____

O _____

action steps for each goal:

O _____ O _____ O _____

O _____ O _____ O _____

O _____ O _____ O _____

fun, relaxation & adventure for today:

O _____

O _____

O _____

evening reflections

- ◯ morning intentions
- ◯ home-cooked food (__x)
- ◯ mindful eating
- ◯ reduced one food
- ◯ tongue scraper
- ◯ hot towel scrub

- ◯ hot water bottle
- ◯ conscious breathing
- ◯ fresh air
- ◯ physical activity
- ◯ prayer/meditation
- ◯ meaningful connections

- ◯ loving work
- ◯ touch/massage
- ◯ laughter
- ◯ time to myself
- ◯ visualized my future
- ◯ quality sleep

high quality nourishment

water/hydrating liquids: _____

whole grains: _____

vegetables: _____

fruits: _____

healthy fats: _____

protein: _____

supplements: _____

how i felt today

mood: _____ digestion: _____

energy: _____ cravings: _____

today i appreciate myself for: _____

_____

choices that did not serve me or support me: _____

_____

today i added in or crowded out: _____

_____

loving thought before bed: _____

_____

morning intentions

date: _____

morning thoughts, feelings & intuitions: _____

_____

_____

_____

i am grateful for: _____

_____

_____

_____

goals for today:

○ _____

○ _____

○ _____

action steps for each goal:

○ _____ ○ _____ ○ _____

○ _____ ○ _____ ○ _____

○ _____ ○ _____ ○ _____

fun, relaxation & adventure for today:

○ _____

○ _____

○ _____

evening reflections

○ morning intentions
○ home-cooked food (__x)
○ mindful eating
○ reduced one food
○ tongue scraper
○ hot towel scrub

○ hot water bottle
○ conscious breathing
○ fresh air
○ physical activity
○ prayer/meditation
○ meaningful connections

○ loving work
○ touch/massage
○ laughter
○ time to myself
○ visualized my future
○ quality sleep

high quality nourishment

water/hydrating liquids: _____

whole grains: _____

vegetables: _____

fruits: _____

healthy fats: _____

protein: _____

supplements: _____

how i felt today

mood: _____ digestion: _____

energy: _____ cravings: _____

today i appreciate myself for: _____

_____

choices that did not serve me or support me: _____

_____

today i added in or crowded out: _____

_____

loving thought before bed: _____

_____

morning intentions

date: _____

morning thoughts, feelings & intuitions: _____

_____

_____

_____

i am grateful for: _____

_____

_____

_____

goals for today:

○ _____

○ _____

○ _____

action steps for each goal:

○ _____ ○ _____ ○ _____

○ _____ ○ _____ ○ _____

○ _____ ○ _____ ○ _____

fun, relaxation & adventure for today:

○ _____

○ _____

○ _____

evening reflections

- ◯ morning intentions
- ◯ home-cooked food (__x)
- ◯ mindful eating
- ◯ reduced one food
- ◯ tongue scraper
- ◯ hot towel scrub

- ◯ hot water bottle
- ◯ conscious breathing
- ◯ fresh air
- ◯ physical activity
- ◯ prayer/meditation
- ◯ meaningful connections

- ◯ loving work
- ◯ touch/massage
- ◯ laughter
- ◯ time to myself
- ◯ visualized my future
- ◯ quality sleep

high quality nourishment

water/hydrating liquids: _____

whole grains: _____

vegetables: _____

fruits: _____

healthy fats: _____

protein: _____

supplements: _____

how i felt today

mood: _____ digestion: _____

energy: _____ cravings: _____

today i appreciate myself for: _____

_____

choices that did not serve me or support me: _____

_____

today i added in or crowded out: _____

_____

loving thought before bed: _____

_____

morning intentions

date: _____

morning thoughts, feelings & intuitions: _____

_____

_____

_____

i am grateful for: _____

_____

_____

_____

goals for today:

○ _____

○ _____

○ _____

action steps for each goal:

○ _____ ○ _____ ○ _____

○ _____ ○ _____ ○ _____

○ _____ ○ _____ ○ _____

fun, relaxation & adventure for today:

○ _____

○ _____

○ _____

evening reflections

- ○ morning intentions
- ○ home-cooked food (__x)
- ○ mindful eating
- ○ reduced one food
- ○ tongue scraper
- ○ hot towel scrub

- ○ hot water bottle
- ○ conscious breathing
- ○ fresh air
- ○ physical activity
- ○ prayer/meditation
- ○ meaningful connections

- ○ loving work
- ○ touch/massage
- ○ laughter
- ○ time to myself
- ○ visualized my future
- ○ quality sleep

high quality nourishment

water/hydrating liquids: _____

whole grains: _____

vegetables: _____

fruits: _____

healthy fats: _____

protein: _____

supplements: _____

how i felt today

mood: _____ digestion: _____

energy: _____ cravings: _____

today i appreciate myself for: _____

_____

choices that did not serve me or support me: _____

_____

today i added in or crowded out: _____

_____

loving thought before bed: _____

_____

morning intentions

date: _____

morning thoughts, feelings & intuitions: _____

_____

_____

_____

i am grateful for: _____

_____

_____

_____

goals for today:

○ _____

○ _____

○ _____

action steps for each goal:

○ _____ ○ _____ ○ _____

○ _____ ○ _____ ○ _____

○ _____ ○ _____ ○ _____

fun, relaxation & adventure for today:

○ _____

○ _____

○ _____

evening reflections

- ○ morning intentions
- ○ home-cooked food (__x)
- ○ mindful eating
- ○ reduced one food
- ○ tongue scraper
- ○ hot towel scrub

- ○ hot water bottle
- ○ conscious breathing
- ○ fresh air
- ○ physical activity
- ○ prayer/meditation
- ○ meaningful connections

- ○ loving work
- ○ touch/massage
- ○ laughter
- ○ time to myself
- ○ visualized my future
- ○ quality sleep

high quality nourishment

water/hydrating liquids: _____

whole grains: _____

vegetables: _____

fruits: _____

healthy fats: _____

protein: _____

supplements: _____

how i felt today

mood: _____   digestion: _____

energy: _____   cravings: _____

today i appreciate myself for: _____

_____

choices that did not serve me or support me: _____

_____

today i added in or crowded out: _____

_____

loving thought before bed: _____

_____

morning intentions

date: _____

morning thoughts, feelings & intuitions: _____

_____

_____

_____

i am grateful for: _____

_____

_____

_____

goals for today:

○ _____

○ _____

○ _____

action steps for each goal:

○ _____ ○ _____ ○ _____

○ _____ ○ _____ ○ _____

○ _____ ○ _____ ○ _____

fun, relaxation & adventure for today:

○ _____

○ _____

○ _____

evening reflections

- ◯ morning intentions
- ◯ home-cooked food (__x)
- ◯ mindful eating
- ◯ reduced one food
- ◯ tongue scraper
- ◯ hot towel scrub

- ◯ hot water bottle
- ◯ conscious breathing
- ◯ fresh air
- ◯ physical activity
- ◯ prayer/meditation
- ◯ meaningful connections

- ◯ loving work
- ◯ touch/massage
- ◯ laughter
- ◯ time to myself
- ◯ visualized my future
- ◯ quality sleep

high quality nourishment

water/hydrating liquids: _____

whole grains: _____

vegetables: _____

fruits: _____

healthy fats: _____

protein: _____

supplements: _____

how i felt today

mood: _____ digestion: _____

energy: _____ cravings: _____

today i appreciate myself for: _____

_____

choices that did not serve me or support me: _____

_____

today i added in or crowded out: _____

_____

loving thought before bed: _____

_____

weekly check-in

dates: _____

what's new & good?

energy & vitality: _____
_____

chewing & digestion: _____
_____

cravings & addictions: _____
_____

hair & skin: _____
_____

mouth, teeth & tongue: _____
_____

body shape & weight: _____
_____

posture & breathing: _____
_____

mood & emotions: _____
_____

relating to others: _____
_____

about the week

most nourishing food: _____

_____

best primary food: _____

_____

special person i appreciate: _____

_____

biggest challenge: _____

_____

main health concern: _____

_____

greatest accomplishment: _____

_____

most fun i had: _____

_____

i got clear that i really want to: _____

_____

other thoughts: _____

_____

next week I plan to: _____

_____

guided exercise

where does my time go?

What are the top 3 priorities in your life?

Do you spend most of your time on these things?

List all the activities that eat up your time.
These might include surfing the web, watching tv or doing
too many favors for others.

How could you reorganize your life
so that you spend more time on what is most important to you?

Top 3 Priorities:
  Relationships (Alan, Ben, girls,
  School   Rest of my family)
  Continuing to heal

Yes.

Cooking
Watching TV Shows

Reorganize:

It's all connected: The meals we eat, the foods we grow,
the policies we form, and the impact we have.

Michael Jacobson, PhD

morning intentions

date: _____

morning thoughts, feelings & intuitions: _____
_____
_____
_____

i am grateful for: _____
_____
_____
_____

goals for today:

○ _____
○ _____
○ _____

action steps for each goal:

○ _____ ○ _____ ○ _____
○ _____ ○ _____ ○ _____
○ _____ ○ _____ ○ _____

fun, relaxation & adventure for today:

○ _____
○ _____
○ _____

evening reflections

○ morning intentions
○ home-cooked food (__x)
○ mindful eating
○ reduced one food
○ tongue scraper
○ hot towel scrub

○ hot water bottle
○ conscious breathing
○ fresh air
○ physical activity
○ prayer/meditation
○ meaningful connections

○ loving work
○ touch/massage
○ laughter
○ time to myself
○ visualized my future
○ quality sleep

high quality nourishment

water/hydrating liquids: _____

whole grains: _____

vegetables: _____

fruits: _____

healthy fats: _____

protein: _____

supplements: _____

how i felt today

mood: _____   digestion: _____

energy: _____   cravings: _____

today i appreciate myself for: _____

_____

choices that did not serve me or support me: _____

_____

today i added in or crowded out: _____

_____

loving thought before bed: _____

_____

morning intentions

date: _____

morning thoughts, feelings & intuitions: _____

_____

_____

_____

i am grateful for: _____

_____

_____

_____

goals for today:

○ _____

○ _____

○ _____

action steps for each goal:

○ _____ ○ _____ ○ _____

○ _____ ○ _____ ○ _____

○ _____ ○ _____ ○ _____

fun, relaxation & adventure for today:

○ _____

○ _____

○ _____

evening reflections

- ⭕ morning intentions
- ⭕ home-cooked food (__x)
- ⭕ mindful eating
- ⭕ reduced one food
- ⭕ tongue scraper
- ⭕ hot towel scrub

- ⭕ hot water bottle
- ⭕ conscious breathing
- ⭕ fresh air
- ⭕ physical activity
- ⭕ prayer/meditation
- ⭕ meaningful connections

- ⭕ loving work
- ⭕ touch/massage
- ⭕ laughter
- ⭕ time to myself
- ⭕ visualized my future
- ⭕ quality sleep

high quality nourishment

water/hydrating liquids: _____

whole grains: _____

vegetables: _____

fruits: _____

healthy fats: _____

protein: _____

supplements: _____

how i felt today

mood: _____   digestion: _____

energy: _____   cravings: _____

today i appreciate myself for: _____

_____

choices that did not serve me or support me: _____

_____

today i added in or crowded out: _____

_____

loving thought before bed: _____

_____

morning intentions

date: _____

morning thoughts, feelings & intuitions: _____

_____

_____

_____

i am grateful for: _____

_____

_____

_____

goals for today:

○ _____

○ _____

○ _____

action steps for each goal:

○ _____ ○ _____ ○ _____

○ _____ ○ _____ ○ _____

○ _____ ○ _____ ○ _____

fun, relaxation & adventure for today:

○ _____

○ _____

○ _____

evening reflections

○ morning intentions
○ home-cooked food (__x)
○ mindful eating
○ reduced one food
○ tongue scraper
○ hot towel scrub

○ hot water bottle
○ conscious breathing
○ fresh air
○ physical activity
○ prayer/meditation
○ meaningful connections

○ loving work
○ touch/massage
○ laughter
○ time to myself
○ visualized my future
○ quality sleep

high quality nourishment

water/hydrating liquids: _____

whole grains: _____

vegetables: _____

fruits: _____

healthy fats: _____

protein: _____

supplements: _____

how i felt today

mood: _____ digestion: _____

energy: _____ cravings: _____

today i appreciate myself for: _____

_____

choices that did not serve me or support me: _____

_____

today i added in or crowded out: _____

_____

loving thought before bed: _____

_____

morning intentions

date: _____

morning thoughts, feelings & intuitions: _____

_____

_____

_____

i am grateful for: _____

_____

_____

_____

goals for today:

○ _____

○ _____

○ _____

action steps for each goal:

○ _____ ○ _____ ○ _____

○ _____ ○ _____ ○ _____

○ _____ ○ _____ ○ _____

fun, relaxation & adventure for today:

○ _____

○ _____

○ _____

evening reflections

○ morning intentions ○ hot water bottle ○ loving work
○ home-cooked food (__x) ○ conscious breathing ○ touch/massage
○ mindful eating ○ fresh air ○ laughter
○ reduced one food ○ physical activity ○ time to myself
○ tongue scraper ○ prayer/meditation ○ visualized my future
○ hot towel scrub ○ meaningful connections ○ quality sleep

high quality nourishment

water/hydrating liquids: _____

whole grains: _____

vegetables: _____

fruits: _____

healthy fats: _____

protein: _____

supplements: _____

how i felt today

mood: _____ digestion: _____

energy: _____ cravings: _____

today i appreciate myself for: _____

_____

choices that did not serve me or support me: _____

_____

today i added in or crowded out: _____

_____

loving thought before bed: _____

_____

morning intentions

date: _____

morning thoughts, feelings & intuitions: _____
_____
_____
_____

i am grateful for: _____
_____
_____
_____

goals for today:

○ _____
○ _____
○ _____

action steps for each goal:

○ _____ ○ _____ ○ _____
○ _____ ○ _____ ○ _____
○ _____ ○ _____ ○ _____

fun, relaxation & adventure for today:

○ _____
○ _____
○ _____

evening reflections

○ morning intentions   ○ hot water bottle   ○ loving work
○ home-cooked food (__x) ○ conscious breathing   ○ touch/massage
○ mindful eating   ○ fresh air   ○ laughter
○ reduced one food   ○ physical activity   ○ time to myself
○ tongue scraper   ○ prayer/meditation   ○ visualized my future
○ hot towel scrub   ○ meaningful connections   ○ quality sleep

high quality nourishment

water/hydrating liquids: _____

whole grains: _____

vegetables: _____

fruits: _____

healthy fats: _____

protein: _____

supplements: _____

how i felt today

mood: _____   digestion: _____

energy: _____   cravings: _____

today i appreciate myself for: _____

_____

choices that did not serve me or support me: _____

_____

today i added in or crowded out: _____

_____

loving thought before bed: _____

_____

morning intentions

date: _____

morning thoughts, feelings & intuitions: _____

_____

_____

_____

i am grateful for: _____

_____

_____

_____

goals for today:

○ _____

○ _____

○ _____

action steps for each goal:

○ _____ ○ _____ ○ _____

○ _____ ○ _____ ○ _____

○ _____ ○ _____ ○ _____

fun, relaxation & adventure for today:

○ _____

○ _____

○ _____

evening reflections

○ morning intentions   ○ hot water bottle   ○ loving work
○ home-cooked food (__x) ○ conscious breathing ○ touch/massage
○ mindful eating   ○ fresh air   ○ laughter
○ reduced one food   ○ physical activity   ○ time to myself
○ tongue scraper   ○ prayer/meditation   ○ visualized my future
○ hot towel scrub   ○ meaningful connections ○ quality sleep

high quality nourishment

water/hydrating liquids: _____

whole grains: _____

vegetables: _____

fruits: _____

healthy fats: _____

protein: _____

supplements: _____

how i felt today

mood: _____ digestion: _____

energy: _____ cravings: _____

today i appreciate myself for: _____

_____

choices that did not serve me or support me: _____

_____

today i added in or crowded out: _____

_____

loving thought before bed: _____

_____

morning intentions

date: _____

morning thoughts, feelings & intuitions: _____

_____

_____

_____

i am grateful for: _____

_____

_____

_____

goals for today:

○ _____

○ _____

○ _____

action steps for each goal:

○ _____ ○ _____ ○ _____

○ _____ ○ _____ ○ _____

○ _____ ○ _____ ○ _____

fun, relaxation & adventure for today:

○ _____

○ _____

○ _____

evening reflections

○ morning intentions
○ home-cooked food (__x)
○ mindful eating
○ reduced one food
○ tongue scraper
○ hot towel scrub

○ hot water bottle
○ conscious breathing
○ fresh air
○ physical activity
○ prayer/meditation
○ meaningful connections

○ loving work
○ touch/massage
○ laughter
○ time to myself
○ visualized my future
○ quality sleep

high quality nourishment

water/hydrating liquids: _____

whole grains: _____

vegetables: _____

fruits: _____

healthy fats: _____

protein: _____

supplements: _____

how i felt today

mood: _____ digestion: _____

energy: _____ cravings: _____

today i appreciate myself for: _____

_____

choices that did not serve me or support me: _____

_____

today i added in or crowded out: _____

_____

loving thought before bed: _____

_____

weekly check-in

dates: _____

what's new & good?

energy & vitality: _____
_____

chewing & digestion: _____
_____

cravings & addictions: _____
_____

hair & skin: _____
_____

mouth, teeth & tongue: _____
_____

body shape & weight: _____
_____

posture & breathing: _____
_____

mood & emotions: _____
_____

relating to others: _____
_____

about the week

most nourishing food: _____
_____

best primary food: _____
_____

special person i appreciate: _____
_____

biggest challenge: _____
_____

main health concern: _____
_____

greatest accomplishment: _____
_____

most fun i had: _____
_____

i got clear that i really want to: _____
_____

other thoughts: _____
_____

next week I plan to: _____
_____

guided exercise

my accomplishments

What are the top 10 things that you have accomplished
so far in your life that you are most proud of?

Make no mistake about it; food is a powerful drug.
In fact, it may be the most powerful drug you will ever take.

Barry Sears, PhD

morning intentions

date: _____

morning thoughts, feelings & intuitions: _____

_____

_____

_____

i am grateful for: _____

_____

_____

_____

goals for today:

○ _____

○ _____

○ _____

action steps for each goal:

○ _____ ○ _____ ○ _____

○ _____ ○ _____ ○ _____

○ _____ ○ _____ ○ _____

fun, relaxation & adventure for today:

○ _____

○ _____

○ _____

evening reflections

○ morning intentions   ○ hot water bottle   ○ loving work
○ home-cooked food (__x) ○ conscious breathing   ○ touch/massage
○ mindful eating   ○ fresh air   ○ laughter
○ reduced one food   ○ physical activity   ○ time to myself
○ tongue scraper   ○ prayer/meditation   ○ visualized my future
○ hot towel scrub   ○ meaningful connections ○ quality sleep

high quality nourishment

water/hydrating liquids: _____

whole grains: _____

vegetables: _____

fruits: _____

healthy fats: _____

protein: _____

supplements: _____

how i felt today

mood: _____ digestion: _____

energy: _____ cravings: _____

today i appreciate myself for: _____

_____

choices that did not serve me or support me: _____

_____

today i added in or crowded out: _____

_____

loving thought before bed: _____

_____

morning intentions

date: _____

morning thoughts, feelings & intuitions: _____
_____
_____
_____

i am grateful for: _____
_____
_____
_____

goals for today:

○ _____
○ _____
○ _____

action steps for each goal:

○ _____ ○ _____ ○ _____
○ _____ ○ _____ ○ _____
○ _____ ○ _____ ○ _____

fun, relaxation & adventure for today:

○ _____
○ _____
○ _____

e v e n i n g   r e f l e c t i o n s

○ morning intentions
○ home-cooked food (__x)
○ mindful eating
○ reduced one food
○ tongue scraper
○ hot towel scrub

○ hot water bottle
○ conscious breathing
○ fresh air
○ physical activity
○ prayer/meditation
○ meaningful connections

○ loving work
○ touch/massage
○ laughter
○ time to myself
○ visualized my future
○ quality sleep

high quality nourishment

water/hydrating liquids: _____

whole grains: _____

vegetables: _____

fruits: _____

healthy fats: _____

protein: _____

supplements: _____

how i felt today

mood: _____ digestion: _____

energy: _____ cravings: _____

today i appreciate myself for: _____

_____

choices that did not serve me or support me: _____

_____

today i added in or crowded out: _____

_____

loving thought before bed: _____

_____

morning intentions

date: _____

morning thoughts, feelings & intuitions: _____
_____
_____
_____

i am grateful for: _____
_____
_____
_____

goals for today:

○ _____
○ _____
○ _____

action steps for each goal:

○ _____ ○ _____ ○ _____
○ _____ ○ _____ ○ _____
○ _____ ○ _____ ○ _____

fun, relaxation & adventure for today:

○ _____
○ _____
○ _____

evening reflections

- ○ morning intentions
- ○ home-cooked food (__x)
- ○ mindful eating
- ○ reduced one food
- ○ tongue scraper
- ○ hot towel scrub

- ○ hot water bottle
- ○ conscious breathing
- ○ fresh air
- ○ physical activity
- ○ prayer/meditation
- ○ meaningful connections

- ○ loving work
- ○ touch/massage
- ○ laughter
- ○ time to myself
- ○ visualized my future
- ○ quality sleep

high quality nourishment

water/hydrating liquids: _____

whole grains: _____

vegetables: _____

fruits: _____

healthy fats: _____

protein: _____

supplements: _____

how i felt today

mood: _____ digestion: _____

energy: _____ cravings: _____

today i appreciate myself for: _____

_____

choices that did not serve me or support me: _____

_____

today i added in or crowded out: _____

_____

loving thought before bed: _____

_____

morning intentions

date: _____

morning thoughts, feelings & intuitions: _____
_____
_____
_____

i am grateful for: _____
_____
_____
_____

goals for today:

○ _____
○ _____
○ _____

action steps for each goal:

○ _____ ○ _____ ○ _____
○ _____ ○ _____ ○ _____
○ _____ ○ _____ ○ _____

fun, relaxation & adventure for today:

○ _____
○ _____
○ _____

evening reflections

- ○ morning intentions
- ○ home-cooked food (__x)
- ○ mindful eating
- ○ reduced one food
- ○ tongue scraper
- ○ hot towel scrub

- ○ hot water bottle
- ○ conscious breathing
- ○ fresh air
- ○ physical activity
- ○ prayer/meditation
- ○ meaningful connections

- ○ loving work
- ○ touch/massage
- ○ laughter
- ○ time to myself
- ○ visualized my future
- ○ quality sleep

high quality nourishment

water/hydrating liquids: _____

whole grains: _____

vegetables: _____

fruits: _____

healthy fats: _____

protein: _____

supplements: _____

how i felt today

mood: _____ digestion: _____

energy: _____ cravings: _____

today i appreciate myself for: _____

_____

choices that did not serve me or support me: _____

_____

today i added in or crowded out: _____

_____

loving thought before bed: _____

_____

morning intentions

date: _____

morning thoughts, feelings & intuitions: _____

_____

_____

_____

i am grateful for: _____

_____

_____

_____

goals for today:

○ _____

○ _____

○ _____

action steps for each goal:

○ _____ ○ _____ ○ _____

○ _____ ○ _____ ○ _____

○ _____ ○ _____ ○ _____

fun, relaxation & adventure for today:

○ _____

○ _____

○ _____

evening reflections

○ morning intentions
○ home-cooked food (__x)
○ mindful eating
○ reduced one food
○ tongue scraper
○ hot towel scrub

○ hot water bottle
○ conscious breathing
○ fresh air
○ physical activity
○ prayer/meditation
○ meaningful connections

○ loving work
○ touch/massage
○ laughter
○ time to myself
○ visualized my future
○ quality sleep

high quality nourishment

water/hydrating liquids: _____

whole grains: _____

vegetables: _____

fruits: _____

healthy fats: _____

protein: _____

supplements: _____

how i felt today

mood: _____ digestion: _____

energy: _____ cravings: _____

today i appreciate myself for: _____

_____

choices that did not serve me or support me: _____

_____

today i added in or crowded out: _____

_____

loving thought before bed: _____

_____

morning intentions

date: _____

morning thoughts, feelings & intuitions: _____

_____

_____

_____

i am grateful for: _____

_____

_____

_____

goals for today:

○ _____

○ _____

○ _____

action steps for each goal:

○ _____   ○ _____   ○ _____

○ _____   ○ _____   ○ _____

○ _____   ○ _____   ○ _____

fun, relaxation & adventure for today:

○ _____

○ _____

○ _____

evening reflections

○ morning intentions
○ home-cooked food (__x)
○ mindful eating
○ reduced one food
○ tongue scraper
○ hot towel scrub

○ hot water bottle
○ conscious breathing
○ fresh air
○ physical activity
○ prayer/meditation
○ meaningful connections

○ loving work
○ touch/massage
○ laughter
○ time to myself
○ visualized my future
○ quality sleep

high quality nourishment

water/hydrating liquids: _____

whole grains: _____

vegetables: _____

fruits: _____

healthy fats: _____

protein: _____

supplements: _____

how i felt today

mood: _____ digestion: _____

energy: _____ cravings: _____

today i appreciate myself for: _____

_____

choices that did not serve me or support me: _____

_____

today i added in or crowded out: _____

_____

loving thought before bed: _____

_____

morning intentions

date: _____

morning thoughts, feelings & intuitions: _____
_____
_____
_____

i am grateful for: _____
_____
_____
_____

goals for today:

○ _____
○ _____
○ _____

action steps for each goal:

○ _____ ○ _____ ○ _____
○ _____ ○ _____ ○ _____
○ _____ ○ _____ ○ _____

fun, relaxation & adventure for today:

○ _____
○ _____
○ _____

evening reflections

○ morning intentions
○ home-cooked food (__x)
○ mindful eating
○ reduced one food
○ tongue scraper
○ hot towel scrub

○ hot water bottle
○ conscious breathing
○ fresh air
○ physical activity
○ prayer/meditation
○ meaningful connections

○ loving work
○ touch/massage
○ laughter
○ time to myself
○ visualized my future
○ quality sleep

high quality nourishment

water/hydrating liquids: _____

whole grains: _____

vegetables: _____

fruits: _____

healthy fats: _____

protein: _____

supplements: _____

how i felt today

mood: _____ digestion: _____

energy: _____ cravings: _____

today i appreciate myself for: _____

_____

choices that did not serve me or support me: _____

_____

today i added in or crowded out: _____

_____

loving thought before bed: _____

_____

weekly check-in

dates: _____

what's new & good?

energy & vitality: _____
_____

chewing & digestion: _____
_____

cravings & addictions: _____
_____

hair & skin: _____
_____

mouth, teeth & tongue: _____
_____

body shape & weight: _____
_____

posture & breathing: _____
_____

mood & emotions: _____
_____

relating to others: _____
_____

about the week

most nourishing food: _____
_____

best primary food: _____
_____

special person i appreciate: _____
_____

biggest challenge: _____
_____

main health concern: _____
_____

greatest accomplishment: _____
_____

most fun i had: _____
_____

i got clear that i really want to: _____
_____

other thoughts: _____
_____

next week I plan to: _____
_____

guided exercise

dream house

Describe your perfect home.

Where is it located?

What is the furniture and decor like?

What kind of a view do you have?

Who lives there with you?

True beauty comes from the inside out.
It emerges from proper thinking, as well as proper nutrition and exercise.

David Wolfe

morning intentions

date: _____

morning thoughts, feelings & intuitions: _____

_____

_____

_____

i am grateful for: _____

_____

_____

_____

goals for today:

○ _____

○ _____

○ _____

action steps for each goal:

○ _____ ○ _____ ○ _____

○ _____ ○ _____ ○ _____

○ _____ ○ _____ ○ _____

fun, relaxation & adventure for today:

○ _____

○ _____

○ _____

evening reflections

- ○ morning intentions
- ○ home-cooked food (__x)
- ○ mindful eating
- ○ reduced one food
- ○ tongue scraper
- ○ hot towel scrub

- ○ hot water bottle
- ○ conscious breathing
- ○ fresh air
- ○ physical activity
- ○ prayer/meditation
- ○ meaningful connections

- ○ loving work
- ○ touch/massage
- ○ laughter
- ○ time to myself
- ○ visualized my future
- ○ quality sleep

high quality nourishment

water/hydrating liquids: _____

whole grains: _____

vegetables: _____

fruits: _____

healthy fats: _____

protein: _____

supplements: _____

how i felt today

mood: _____   digestion: _____

energy: _____   cravings: _____

today i appreciate myself for: _____

_____

choices that did not serve me or support me: _____

_____

today i added in or crowded out: _____

_____

loving thought before bed: _____

_____

morning intentions

date: _____

morning thoughts, feelings & intuitions: _____

_____

_____

_____

i am grateful for: _____

_____

_____

_____

goals for today:

○ _____

○ _____

○ _____

action steps for each goal:

○ _____ ○ _____ ○ _____

○ _____ ○ _____ ○ _____

○ _____ ○ _____ ○ _____

fun, relaxation & adventure for today:

○ _____

○ _____

○ _____

evening reflections

- ○ morning intentions
- ○ home-cooked food (__x)
- ○ mindful eating
- ○ reduced one food
- ○ tongue scraper
- ○ hot towel scrub

- ○ hot water bottle
- ○ conscious breathing
- ○ fresh air
- ○ physical activity
- ○ prayer/meditation
- ○ meaningful connections

- ○ loving work
- ○ touch/massage
- ○ laughter
- ○ time to myself
- ○ visualized my future
- ○ quality sleep

high quality nourishment

water/hydrating liquids: _____

whole grains: _____

vegetables: _____

fruits: _____

healthy fats: _____

protein: _____

supplements: _____

how i felt today

mood: _____   digestion: _____

energy: _____   cravings: _____

today i appreciate myself for: _____

_____

choices that did not serve me or support me: _____

_____

today i added in or crowded out: _____

_____

loving thought before bed: _____

_____

morning intentions

date: _____

morning thoughts, feelings & intuitions: _____

_____

_____

_____

i am grateful for: _____

_____

_____

_____

goals for today:

O _____

O _____

O _____

action steps for each goal:

O _____ O _____ O _____

O _____ O _____ O _____

O _____ O _____ O _____

fun, relaxation & adventure for today:

O _____

O _____

O _____

evening reflections

○ morning intentions
○ home-cooked food (__x)
○ mindful eating
○ reduced one food
○ tongue scraper
○ hot towel scrub

○ hot water bottle
○ conscious breathing
○ fresh air
○ physical activity
○ prayer/meditation
○ meaningful connections

○ loving work
○ touch/massage
○ laughter
○ time to myself
○ visualized my future
○ quality sleep

high quality nourishment

water/hydrating liquids: _____

whole grains: _____

vegetables: _____

fruits: _____

healthy fats: _____

protein: _____

supplements: _____

how i felt today

mood: _____ digestion: _____

energy: _____ cravings: _____

today i appreciate myself for: _____

_____

choices that did not serve me or support me: _____

_____

today i added in or crowded out: _____

_____

loving thought before bed: _____

_____

morning intentions

date: _____

morning thoughts, feelings & intuitions: _____

_____

_____

_____

i am grateful for: _____

_____

_____

_____

goals for today:

○ _____

○ _____

○ _____

action steps for each goal:

○ _____   ○ _____   ○ _____

○ _____   ○ _____   ○ _____

○ _____   ○ _____   ○ _____

fun, relaxation & adventure for today:

○ _____

○ _____

○ _____

evening reflections

○ morning intentions   ○ hot water bottle   ○ loving work
○ home-cooked food (__x)   ○ conscious breathing   ○ touch/massage
○ mindful eating   ○ fresh air   ○ laughter
○ reduced one food   ○ physical activity   ○ time to myself
○ tongue scraper   ○ prayer/meditation   ○ visualized my future
○ hot towel scrub   ○ meaningful connections   ○ quality sleep

high quality nourishment

water/hydrating liquids: _____

whole grains: _____

vegetables: _____

fruits: _____

healthy fats: _____

protein: _____

supplements: _____

how i felt today

mood: _____ digestion: _____

energy: _____ cravings: _____

today i appreciate myself for: _____

_____

choices that did not serve me or support me: _____

_____

today i added in or crowded out: _____

_____

loving thought before bed: _____

_____

morning intentions

date: _____

morning thoughts, feelings & intuitions: _____

_____

_____

_____

i am grateful for: _____

_____

_____

_____

goals for today:

○ _____

○ _____

○ _____

action steps for each goal:

○ _____ ○ _____ ○ _____

○ _____ ○ _____ ○ _____

○ _____ ○ _____ ○ _____

fun, relaxation & adventure for today:

○ _____

○ _____

○ _____

evening reflections

○ morning intentions
○ home-cooked food (__x)
○ mindful eating
○ reduced one food
○ tongue scraper
○ hot towel scrub

○ hot water bottle
○ conscious breathing
○ fresh air
○ physical activity
○ prayer/meditation
○ meaningful connections

○ loving work
○ touch/massage
○ laughter
○ time to myself
○ visualized my future
○ quality sleep

high quality nourishment

water/hydrating liquids: _____

whole grains: _____

vegetables: _____

fruits: _____

healthy fats: _____

protein: _____

supplements: _____

how i felt today

mood: _____   digestion: _____

energy: _____   cravings: _____

today i appreciate myself for: _____

_____

choices that did not serve me or support me: _____

_____

today i added in or crowded out: _____

_____

loving thought before bed: _____

_____

morning intentions

date: _____

morning thoughts, feelings & intuitions: _____

_____

_____

_____

i am grateful for: _____

_____

_____

_____

goals for today:

○ _____

○ _____

○ _____

action steps for each goal:

○ _____ ○ _____ ○ _____

○ _____ ○ _____ ○ _____

○ _____ ○ _____ ○ _____

fun, relaxation & adventure for today:

○ _____

○ _____

○ _____

evening reflections

○ morning intentions ○ hot water bottle ○ loving work
○ home-cooked food (__x) ○ conscious breathing ○ touch/massage
○ mindful eating ○ fresh air ○ laughter
○ reduced one food ○ physical activity ○ time to myself
○ tongue scraper ○ prayer/meditation ○ visualized my future
○ hot towel scrub ○ meaningful connections ○ quality sleep

high quality nourishment

water/hydrating liquids: _____

whole grains: _____

vegetables: _____

fruits: _____

healthy fats: _____

protein: _____

supplements: _____

how i felt today

mood: _____ digestion: _____

energy: _____ cravings: _____

today i appreciate myself for: _____

_____

choices that did not serve me or support me: _____

_____

today i added in or crowded out: _____

_____

loving thought before bed: _____

_____

morning intentions

date: _____

morning thoughts, feelings & intuitions: _____

_____

_____

_____

i am grateful for: _____

_____

_____

_____

goals for today:

○ _____

○ _____

○ _____

action steps for each goal:

○ _____ ○ _____ ○ _____

○ _____ ○ _____ ○ _____

○ _____ ○ _____ ○ _____

fun, relaxation & adventure for today:

○ _____

○ _____

○ _____

evening reflections

- ○ morning intentions
- ○ home-cooked food (__x)
- ○ mindful eating
- ○ reduced one food
- ○ tongue scraper
- ○ hot towel scrub

- ○ hot water bottle
- ○ conscious breathing
- ○ fresh air
- ○ physical activity
- ○ prayer/meditation
- ○ meaningful connections

- ○ loving work
- ○ touch/massage
- ○ laughter
- ○ time to myself
- ○ visualized my future
- ○ quality sleep

high quality nourishment

water/hydrating liquids: _____

whole grains: _____

vegetables: _____

fruits: _____

healthy fats: _____

protein: _____

supplements: _____

how i felt today

mood: _____ digestion: _____

energy: _____ cravings: _____

today i appreciate myself for: _____

_____

choices that did not serve me or support me: _____

_____

today i added in or crowded out: _____

_____

loving thought before bed: _____

_____

month two progress

dates: _____

what's changed this month?

food & cooking: _____
_____
_____

self-care: _____
_____
_____

physical health: _____
_____
_____

main health concern: _____
_____
_____

habits, cravings & addictions: _____
_____
_____

moods, thoughts & feelings: _____
_____
_____

primary food progress

career: _____

_____

relationships: _____

_____

physical activity: _____

_____

spirituality: _____

_____

creativity: _____

_____

fun, relaxation & adventure: _____

_____

other accomplishments: _____

_____

_____

_____

_____

_____

No single food will make or break good health. But the kinds
of foods you choose day in and day out have a major impact.

Walter Willett, MD

You are not creating a new you;
you are releasing a hidden you.
The process is one of self-discovery.
The hidden you that wants to emerge
is in perfect balance.

Deepak Chopra, MD

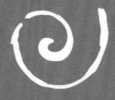

month three

circle of life

This exercise will help you discover which primary foods need attention in order for you to create more balance in your life. The circle has twelve sections. Place a dot on the line for each section to designate how satisfied you are with that aspect of your life. A dot placed towards the center of the circle indicates dissatisfaction, while a dot placed towards the periphery indicates ultimate happiness. When you have placed a dot on each line, connect the dots to see your Circle of Life. Now you have a clear visual of any areas that may need your attention. You will complete this exercise again next month to see if your circle has become more balanced.

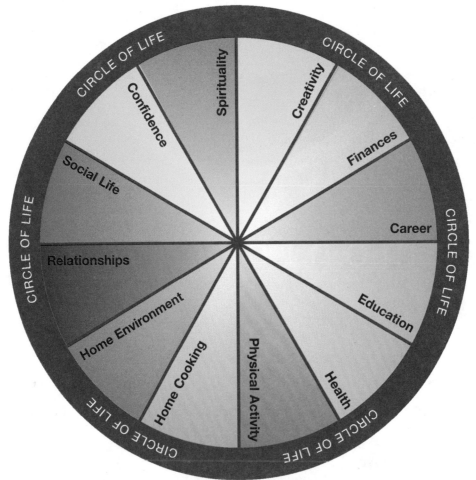

wish list

Now that you have identified areas of your life that are out of balance or unsatisfying, what would it take to bring them into balance? What experiences, items, relationships or feelings would make those parts of your life juicy and exciting? This exercise will help you get in touch with your desires. In the table below, begin listing simple and obvious wishes. Bigger, more exciting desires will come as you write.

Keep these desires in mind when setting your morning intentions. Whenever you fulfill a desire, put an X in the "done" column. In the "gratitude" column, thank anyone who may have helped. You might be thanking yourself. Notice how, as you take better care of yourself, your desires naturally come true, and your life becomes more fulfilling.

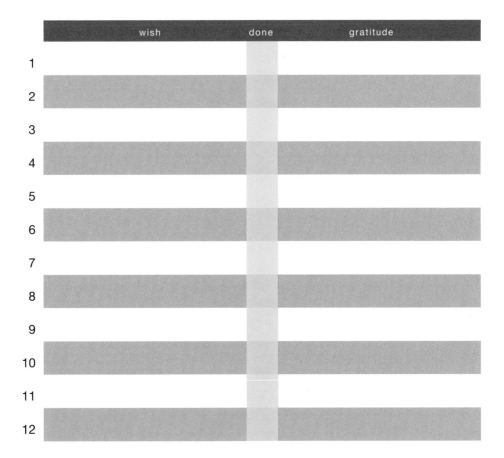

	wish	done	gratitude
1			
2			
3			
4			
5			
6			
7			
8			
9			
10			
11			
12			

morning intentions

date: _____

morning thoughts, feelings & intuitions: _____

_____

_____

_____

i am grateful for: _____

_____

_____

_____

goals for today:

○ _____

○ _____

○ _____

action steps for each goal:

○ _____ ○ _____ ○ _____

○ _____ ○ _____ ○ _____

○ _____ ○ _____ ○ _____

fun, relaxation & adventure for today:

○ _____

○ _____

○ _____

evening reflections

- ○ morning intentions
- ○ home-cooked food (__x)
- ○ mindful eating
- ○ reduced one food
- ○ tongue scraper
- ○ hot towel scrub

- ○ hot water bottle
- ○ conscious breathing
- ○ fresh air
- ○ physical activity
- ○ prayer/meditation
- ○ meaningful connections

- ○ loving work
- ○ touch/massage
- ○ laughter
- ○ time to myself
- ○ visualized my future
- ○ quality sleep

high quality nourishment

water/hydrating liquids: _____

whole grains: _____

vegetables: _____

fruits: _____

healthy fats: _____

protein: _____

supplements: _____

how i felt today

mood: _____ digestion: _____

energy: _____ cravings: _____

today i appreciate myself for: _____

_____

choices that did not serve me or support me: _____

_____

today i added in or crowded out: _____

_____

loving thought before bed: _____

_____

morning intentions

date: _____

morning thoughts, feelings & intuitions: _____

_____

_____

_____

i am grateful for: _____

_____

_____

_____

goals for today:

○ _____

○ _____

○ _____

action steps for each goal:

○ _____ ○ _____ ○ _____

○ _____ ○ _____ ○ _____

○ _____ ○ _____ ○ _____

fun, relaxation & adventure for today:

○ _____

○ _____

○ _____

evening reflections

○ morning intentions
○ home-cooked food (__x)
○ mindful eating
○ reduced one food
○ tongue scraper
○ hot towel scrub

○ hot water bottle
○ conscious breathing
○ fresh air
○ physical activity
○ prayer/meditation
○ meaningful connections

○ loving work
○ touch/massage
○ laughter
○ time to myself
○ visualized my future
○ quality sleep

high quality nourishment

water/hydrating liquids: _____

whole grains: _____

vegetables: _____

fruits: _____

healthy fats: _____

protein: _____

supplements: _____

how i felt today

mood: _____ digestion: _____

energy: _____ cravings: _____

today i appreciate myself for: _____

_____

choices that did not serve me or support me: _____

_____

today i added in or crowded out: _____

_____

loving thought before bed: _____

_____

morning intentions

date: _____

morning thoughts, feelings & intuitions: _____

_____

_____

_____

i am grateful for: _____

_____

_____

_____

goals for today:

○ _____

○ _____

○ _____

action steps for each goal:

○ _____   ○ _____   ○ _____

○ _____   ○ _____   ○ _____

○ _____   ○ _____   ○ _____

fun, relaxation & adventure for today:

○ _____

○ _____

○ _____

evening reflections

○ morning intentions
○ home-cooked food (__x)
○ mindful eating
○ reduced one food
○ tongue scraper
○ hot towel scrub

○ hot water bottle
○ conscious breathing
○ fresh air
○ physical activity
○ prayer/meditation
○ meaningful connections

○ loving work
○ touch/massage
○ laughter
○ time to myself
○ visualized my future
○ quality sleep

high quality nourishment

water/hydrating liquids: _____

whole grains: _____

vegetables: _____

fruits: _____

healthy fats: _____

protein: _____

supplements: _____

how i felt today

mood: _____ digestion: _____

energy: _____ cravings: _____

today i appreciate myself for: _____

_____

choices that did not serve me or support me: _____

_____

today i added in or crowded out: _____

_____

loving thought before bed: _____

_____

morning intentions

date: _____

morning thoughts, feelings & intuitions: _____

_____

_____

_____

i am grateful for: _____

_____

_____

_____

goals for today:

○ _____

○ _____

○ _____

action steps for each goal:

○ _____ ○ _____ ○ _____

○ _____ ○ _____ ○ _____

○ _____ ○ _____ ○ _____

fun, relaxation & adventure for today:

○ _____

○ _____

○ _____

evening reflections

○ morning intentions
○ home-cooked food (__x)
○ mindful eating
○ reduced one food
○ tongue scraper
○ hot towel scrub

○ hot water bottle
○ conscious breathing
○ fresh air
○ physical activity
○ prayer/meditation
○ meaningful connections

○ loving work
○ touch/massage
○ laughter
○ time to myself
○ visualized my future
○ quality sleep

high quality nourishment

water/hydrating liquids: _____

whole grains: _____

vegetables: _____

fruits: _____

healthy fats: _____

protein: _____

supplements: _____

how i felt today

mood: _____ digestion: _____

energy: _____ cravings: _____

today i appreciate myself for: _____

_____

choices that did not serve me or support me: _____

_____

today i added in or crowded out: _____

_____

loving thought before bed: _____

_____

morning intentions

date: _____

morning thoughts, feelings & intuitions: _____

_____

_____

_____

i am grateful for: _____

_____

_____

_____

goals for today:

○ _____

○ _____

○ _____

action steps for each goal:

○ _____ ○ _____ ○ _____

○ _____ ○ _____ ○ _____

○ _____ ○ _____ ○ _____

fun, relaxation & adventure for today:

○ _____

○ _____

○ _____

evening reflections

- ○ morning intentions
- ○ home-cooked food (__x)
- ○ mindful eating
- ○ reduced one food
- ○ tongue scraper
- ○ hot towel scrub

- ○ hot water bottle
- ○ conscious breathing
- ○ fresh air
- ○ physical activity
- ○ prayer/meditation
- ○ meaningful connections

- ○ loving work
- ○ touch/massage
- ○ laughter
- ○ time to myself
- ○ visualized my future
- ○ quality sleep

high quality nourishment

water/hydrating liquids: _____

whole grains: _____

vegetables: _____

fruits: _____

healthy fats: _____

protein: _____

supplements: _____

how i felt today

mood: _____   digestion: _____

energy: _____   cravings: _____

today i appreciate myself for: _____

_____

choices that did not serve me or support me: _____

_____

today i added in or crowded out: _____

_____

loving thought before bed: _____

_____

morning intentions

date: _____

morning thoughts, feelings & intuitions: _____

_____

_____

_____

i am grateful for: _____

_____

_____

_____

goals for today:

○ _____

○ _____

○ _____

action steps for each goal:

○ _____ ○ _____ ○ _____

○ _____ ○ _____ ○ _____

○ _____ ○ _____ ○ _____

fun, relaxation & adventure for today:

○ _____

○ _____

○ _____

evening reflections

○ morning intentions
○ home-cooked food (__x)
○ mindful eating
○ reduced one food
○ tongue scraper
○ hot towel scrub

○ hot water bottle
○ conscious breathing
○ fresh air
○ physical activity
○ prayer/meditation
○ meaningful connections

○ loving work
○ touch/massage
○ laughter
○ time to myself
○ visualized my future
○ quality sleep

high quality nourishment

water/hydrating liquids: _____

whole grains: _____

vegetables: _____

fruits: _____

healthy fats: _____

protein: _____

supplements: _____

how i felt today

mood: _____ digestion: _____

energy: _____ cravings: _____

today i appreciate myself for: _____

_____

choices that did not serve me or support me: _____

_____

today i added in or crowded out: _____

_____

loving thought before bed: _____

_____

morning intentions

date: _____

morning thoughts, feelings & intuitions: _____

_____

_____

_____

i am grateful for: _____

_____

_____

_____

goals for today:

○ _____

○ _____

○ _____

action steps for each goal:

○ _____ ○ _____ ○ _____

○ _____ ○ _____ ○ _____

○ _____ ○ _____ ○ _____

fun, relaxation & adventure for today:

○ _____

○ _____

○ _____

evening reflections

- ◯ morning intentions
- ◯ home-cooked food (__x)
- ◯ mindful eating
- ◯ reduced one food
- ◯ tongue scraper
- ◯ hot towel scrub

- ◯ hot water bottle
- ◯ conscious breathing
- ◯ fresh air
- ◯ physical activity
- ◯ prayer/meditation
- ◯ meaningful connections

- ◯ loving work
- ◯ touch/massage
- ◯ laughter
- ◯ time to myself
- ◯ visualized my future
- ◯ quality sleep

high quality nourishment

water/hydrating liquids: _____

whole grains: _____

vegetables: _____

fruits: _____

healthy fats: _____

protein: _____

supplements: _____

how i felt today

mood: _____ digestion: _____

energy: _____ cravings: _____

today i appreciate myself for: _____

_____

choices that did not serve me or support me: _____

_____

today i added in or crowded out: _____

_____

loving thought before bed: _____

_____

weekly check-in

dates: _____

what's new & good?

energy & vitality: _____
_____

chewing & digestion: _____
_____

cravings & addictions: _____
_____

hair & skin: _____
_____

mouth, teeth & tongue: _____
_____

body shape & weight: _____
_____

posture & breathing: _____
_____

mood & emotions: _____
_____

relating to others: _____
_____

about the week

most nourishing food: _____

_____

best primary food: _____

_____

special person i appreciate: _____

_____

biggest challenge: _____

_____

main health concern: _____

_____

greatest accomplishment: _____

_____

most fun i had: _____

_____

i got clear that i really want to: _____

_____

other thoughts: _____

_____

next week I plan to: _____

_____

guided exercise

unfinished business

List all your unfinished projects that drain your energy
and keep you from focusing on your present and future.
These may include cluttered closets, piles of papers, incomplete
craft projects, degrees and travel plans, or unkept promises.

How can you get these parts of your life cleaned up?

You can't change yesterdays, but you can change tomorrows.

Howard Lyman

morning intentions

date: _____

morning thoughts, feelings & intuitions: _____

_____

_____

_____

i am grateful for: _____

_____

_____

_____

goals for today:

O _____

O _____

O _____

action steps for each goal:

O _____ O _____ O _____

O _____ O _____ O _____

O _____ O _____ O _____

fun, relaxation & adventure for today:

O _____

O _____

O _____

evening reflections

- ○ morning intentions
- ○ home-cooked food (__x)
- ○ mindful eating
- ○ reduced one food
- ○ tongue scraper
- ○ hot towel scrub

- ○ hot water bottle
- ○ conscious breathing
- ○ fresh air
- ○ physical activity
- ○ prayer/meditation
- ○ meaningful connections

- ○ loving work
- ○ touch/massage
- ○ laughter
- ○ time to myself
- ○ visualized my future
- ○ quality sleep

high quality nourishment

water/hydrating liquids: _____

whole grains: _____

vegetables: _____

fruits: _____

healthy fats: _____

protein: _____

supplements: _____

how i felt today

mood: _____ digestion: _____

energy: _____ cravings: _____

today i appreciate myself for: _____

_____

choices that did not serve me or support me: _____

_____

today i added in or crowded out: _____

_____

loving thought before bed: _____

_____

morning intentions

date: _____

morning thoughts, feelings & intuitions: _____

_____

_____

_____

i am grateful for: _____

_____

_____

_____

goals for today:

○ _____

○ _____

○ _____

action steps for each goal:

○ _____ ○ _____ ○ _____

○ _____ ○ _____ ○ _____

○ _____ ○ _____ ○ _____

fun, relaxation & adventure for today:

○ _____

○ _____

○ _____

evening reflections

- ◯ morning intentions
- ◯ home-cooked food (__x)
- ◯ mindful eating
- ◯ reduced one food
- ◯ tongue scraper
- ◯ hot towel scrub

- ◯ hot water bottle
- ◯ conscious breathing
- ◯ fresh air
- ◯ physical activity
- ◯ prayer/meditation
- ◯ meaningful connections

- ◯ loving work
- ◯ touch/massage
- ◯ laughter
- ◯ time to myself
- ◯ visualized my future
- ◯ quality sleep

high quality nourishment

water/hydrating liquids: _____

whole grains: _____

vegetables: _____

fruits: _____

healthy fats: _____

protein: _____

supplements: _____

how i felt today

mood: _____   digestion: _____

energy: _____   cravings: _____

today i appreciate myself for: _____

_____

choices that did not serve me or support me: _____

_____

today i added in or crowded out: _____

_____

loving thought before bed: _____

_____

morning intentions

date: _____

morning thoughts, feelings & intuitions: _____

_____

_____

_____

i am grateful for: _____

_____

_____

_____

goals for today:

○ _____

○ _____

○ _____

action steps for each goal:

○ _____ ○ _____ ○ _____

○ _____ ○ _____ ○ _____

○ _____ ○ _____ ○ _____

fun, relaxation & adventure for today:

○ _____

○ _____

○ _____

evening reflections

○ morning intentions
○ home-cooked food (__x)
○ mindful eating
○ reduced one food
○ tongue scraper
○ hot towel scrub

○ hot water bottle
○ conscious breathing
○ fresh air
○ physical activity
○ prayer/meditation
○ meaningful connections

○ loving work
○ touch/massage
○ laughter
○ time to myself
○ visualized my future
○ quality sleep

high quality nourishment

water/hydrating liquids: _____

whole grains: _____

vegetables: _____

fruits: _____

healthy fats: _____

protein: _____

supplements: _____

how i felt today

mood: _____ digestion: _____

energy: _____ cravings: _____

today i appreciate myself for: _____

_____

choices that did not serve me or support me: _____

_____

today i added in or crowded out: _____

_____

loving thought before bed: _____

_____

morning intentions

date: _____

morning thoughts, feelings & intuitions: _____
_____
_____
_____

i am grateful for: _____
_____
_____
_____

goals for today:

◯ _____
◯ _____
◯ _____

action steps for each goal:

◯ _____ ◯ _____ ◯ _____
◯ _____ ◯ _____ ◯ _____
◯ _____ ◯ _____ ◯ _____

fun, relaxation & adventure for today:

◯ _____
◯ _____
◯ _____

evening reflections

- ○ morning intentions
- ○ home-cooked food (__x)
- ○ mindful eating
- ○ reduced one food
- ○ tongue scraper
- ○ hot towel scrub
- ○ hot water bottle
- ○ conscious breathing
- ○ fresh air
- ○ physical activity
- ○ prayer/meditation
- ○ meaningful connections
- ○ loving work
- ○ touch/massage
- ○ laughter
- ○ time to myself
- ○ visualized my future
- ○ quality sleep

high quality nourishment

water/hydrating liquids: _____

whole grains: _____

vegetables: _____

fruits: _____

healthy fats: _____

protein: _____

supplements: _____

how i felt today

mood: _____   digestion: _____

energy: _____   cravings: _____

today i appreciate myself for: _____

_____

choices that did not serve me or support me: _____

_____

today i added in or crowded out: _____

_____

loving thought before bed: _____

_____

morning intentions

date: _____

morning thoughts, feelings & intuitions: _____

_____

_____

_____

i am grateful for: _____

_____

_____

_____

goals for today:

○ _____

○ _____

○ _____

action steps for each goal:

○ _____ ○ _____ ○ _____

○ _____ ○ _____ ○ _____

○ _____ ○ _____ ○ _____

fun, relaxation & adventure for today:

○ _____

○ _____

○ _____

evening reflections

○ morning intentions
○ home-cooked food (__x)
○ mindful eating
○ reduced one food
○ tongue scraper
○ hot towel scrub

○ hot water bottle
○ conscious breathing
○ fresh air
○ physical activity
○ prayer/meditation
○ meaningful connections

○ loving work
○ touch/massage
○ laughter
○ time to myself
○ visualized my future
○ quality sleep

high quality nourishment

water/hydrating liquids: _____

whole grains: _____

vegetables: _____

fruits: _____

healthy fats: _____

protein: _____

supplements: _____

how i felt today

mood: _____ digestion: _____

energy: _____ cravings: _____

today i appreciate myself for: _____

_____

choices that did not serve me or support me: _____

_____

today i added in or crowded out: _____

_____

loving thought before bed: _____

_____

morning intentions

date: _____

morning thoughts, feelings & intuitions: _____

_____

_____

_____

i am grateful for: _____

_____

_____

_____

goals for today:

○ _____

○ _____

○ _____

action steps for each goal:

○ _____ ○ _____ ○ _____

○ _____ ○ _____ ○ _____

○ _____ ○ _____ ○ _____

fun, relaxation & adventure for today:

○ _____

○ _____

○ _____

evening reflections

○ morning intentions
○ home-cooked food (__x)
○ mindful eating
○ reduced one food
○ tongue scraper
○ hot towel scrub

○ hot water bottle
○ conscious breathing
○ fresh air
○ physical activity
○ prayer/meditation
○ meaningful connections

○ loving work
○ touch/massage
○ laughter
○ time to myself
○ visualized my future
○ quality sleep

high quality nourishment

water/hydrating liquids: _____

whole grains: _____

vegetables: _____

fruits: _____

healthy fats: _____

protein: _____

supplements: _____

how i felt today

mood: _____ digestion: _____

energy: _____ cravings: _____

today i appreciate myself for: _____

_____

choices that did not serve me or support me: _____

_____

today i added in or crowded out: _____

_____

loving thought before bed: _____

_____

morning intentions

date: _____

morning thoughts, feelings & intuitions: _____

_____

_____

_____

i am grateful for: _____

_____

_____

_____

goals for today:

○ _____

○ _____

○ _____

action steps for each goal:

○ _____ ○ _____ ○ _____

○ _____ ○ _____ ○ _____

○ _____ ○ _____ ○ _____

fun, relaxation & adventure for today:

○ _____

○ _____

○ _____

evening reflections

○ morning intentions   ○ hot water bottle   ○ loving work
○ home-cooked food (__x)   ○ conscious breathing   ○ touch/massage
○ mindful eating   ○ fresh air   ○ laughter
○ reduced one food   ○ physical activity   ○ time to myself
○ tongue scraper   ○ prayer/meditation   ○ visualized my future
○ hot towel scrub   ○ meaningful connections   ○ quality sleep

high quality nourishment

water/hydrating liquids: _____

whole grains: _____

vegetables: _____

fruits: _____

healthy fats: _____

protein: _____

supplements: _____

how i felt today

mood: _____   digestion: _____

energy: _____   cravings: _____

today i appreciate myself for: _____

_____

choices that did not serve me or support me: _____

_____

today i added in or crowded out: _____

_____

loving thought before bed: _____

_____

weekly check-in

dates: _____

what's new & good?

energy & vitality: _____
_____

chewing & digestion: _____
_____

cravings & addictions: _____
_____

hair & skin: _____
_____

mouth, teeth & tongue: _____
_____

body shape & weight: _____
_____

posture & breathing: _____
_____

mood & emotions: _____
_____

relating to others: _____
_____

about the week

most nourishing food: _____

_____

best primary food: _____

_____

special person i appreciate: _____

_____

biggest challenge: _____

_____

main health concern: _____

_____

greatest accomplishment: _____

_____

most fun i had: _____

_____

i got clear that i really want to: _____

_____

other thoughts: _____

_____

next week I plan to: _____

_____

guided exercise

champions, mentors and role models

Who are 3 people from your past who positively influenced your life
and helped you become the person you are today?

Who are your champions, mentors and role models today?

What qualities do you love about those people?

Who are some people who you know look up to you?

What do you think they admire and appreciate about you?

Food is a drug. Food is medicine. Hippocrates taught us this centuries ago. Whether it is good or bad medicine depends on how you use it.

Mark Hyman, MD

morning intentions

date: _____

morning thoughts, feelings & intuitions: _____

_____

_____

_____

i am grateful for: _____

_____

_____

_____

goals for today:

○ _____

○ _____

○ _____

action steps for each goal:

○ _____ ○ _____ ○ _____

○ _____ ○ _____ ○ _____

○ _____ ○ _____ ○ _____

fun, relaxation & adventure for today:

○ _____

○ _____

○ _____

evening reflections

- ◯ morning intentions
- ◯ home-cooked food (__x)
- ◯ mindful eating
- ◯ reduced one food
- ◯ tongue scraper
- ◯ hot towel scrub

- ◯ hot water bottle
- ◯ conscious breathing
- ◯ fresh air
- ◯ physical activity
- ◯ prayer/meditation
- ◯ meaningful connections

- ◯ loving work
- ◯ touch/massage
- ◯ laughter
- ◯ time to myself
- ◯ visualized my future
- ◯ quality sleep

high quality nourishment

water/hydrating liquids: _____

whole grains: _____

vegetables: _____

fruits: _____

healthy fats: _____

protein: _____

supplements: _____

how i felt today

mood: _____   digestion: _____

energy: _____   cravings: _____

today i appreciate myself for: _____

_____

choices that did not serve me or support me: _____

_____

today i added in or crowded out: _____

_____

loving thought before bed: _____

_____

morning intentions

date: _____

morning thoughts, feelings & intuitions: _____

_____

_____

_____

i am grateful for: _____

_____

_____

_____

goals for today:

○ _____

○ _____

○ _____

action steps for each goal:

○ _____ ○ _____ ○ _____

○ _____ ○ _____ ○ _____

○ _____ ○ _____ ○ _____

fun, relaxation & adventure for today:

○ _____

○ _____

○ _____

evening reflections

- ○ morning intentions
- ○ home-cooked food (__x)
- ○ mindful eating
- ○ reduced one food
- ○ tongue scraper
- ○ hot towel scrub

- ○ hot water bottle
- ○ conscious breathing
- ○ fresh air
- ○ physical activity
- ○ prayer/meditation
- ○ meaningful connections

- ○ loving work
- ○ touch/massage
- ○ laughter
- ○ time to myself
- ○ visualized my future
- ○ quality sleep

high quality nourishment

water/hydrating liquids: _____

whole grains: _____

vegetables: _____

fruits: _____

healthy fats: _____

protein: _____

supplements: _____

how i felt today

mood: _____ digestion: _____

energy: _____ cravings: _____

today i appreciate myself for: _____

_____

choices that did not serve me or support me: _____

_____

today i added in or crowded out: _____

_____

loving thought before bed: _____

_____

morning intentions

date: _____

morning thoughts, feelings & intuitions: _____

_____

_____

_____

i am grateful for: _____

_____

_____

_____

goals for today:

○ _____

○ _____

○ _____

action steps for each goal:

○ _____ ○ _____ ○ _____

○ _____ ○ _____ ○ _____

○ _____ ○ _____ ○ _____

fun, relaxation & adventure for today:

○ _____

○ _____

○ _____

evening reflections

- ○ morning intentions
- ○ home-cooked food (__x)
- ○ mindful eating
- ○ reduced one food
- ○ tongue scraper
- ○ hot towel scrub

- ○ hot water bottle
- ○ conscious breathing
- ○ fresh air
- ○ physical activity
- ○ prayer/meditation
- ○ meaningful connections

- ○ loving work
- ○ touch/massage
- ○ laughter
- ○ time to myself
- ○ visualized my future
- ○ quality sleep

high quality nourishment

water/hydrating liquids: _____

whole grains: _____

vegetables: _____

fruits: _____

healthy fats: _____

protein: _____

supplements: _____

how i felt today

mood: _____   digestion: _____

energy: _____   cravings: _____

today i appreciate myself for: _____

_____

choices that did not serve me or support me: _____

_____

today i added in or crowded out: _____

_____

loving thought before bed: _____

_____

morning intentions

date: _____

morning thoughts, feelings & intuitions: _____

_____

_____

_____

i am grateful for: _____

_____

_____

_____

goals for today:

○ _____

○ _____

○ _____

action steps for each goal:

○ _____   ○ _____   ○ _____

○ _____   ○ _____   ○ _____

○ _____   ○ _____   ○ _____

fun, relaxation & adventure for today:

○ _____

○ _____

○ _____

evening reflections

○ morning intentions
○ home-cooked food (__x)
○ mindful eating
○ reduced one food
○ tongue scraper
○ hot towel scrub

○ hot water bottle
○ conscious breathing
○ fresh air
○ physical activity
○ prayer/meditation
○ meaningful connections

○ loving work
○ touch/massage
○ laughter
○ time to myself
○ visualized my future
○ quality sleep

high quality nourishment

water/hydrating liquids: _____

whole grains: _____

vegetables: _____

fruits: _____

healthy fats: _____

protein: _____

supplements: _____

how i felt today

mood: _____ digestion: _____

energy: _____ cravings: _____

today i appreciate myself for: _____

_____

choices that did not serve me or support me: _____

_____

today i added in or crowded out: _____

_____

loving thought before bed: _____

_____

morning intentions

date: _____

morning thoughts, feelings & intuitions: _____

_____

_____

_____

i am grateful for: _____

_____

_____

_____

goals for today:

○ _____

○ _____

○ _____

action steps for each goal:

○ _____ ○ _____ ○ _____

○ _____ ○ _____ ○ _____

○ _____ ○ _____ ○ _____

fun, relaxation & adventure for today:

○ _____

○ _____

○ _____

evening reflections

- ◯ morning intentions
- ◯ home-cooked food (__x)
- ◯ mindful eating
- ◯ reduced one food
- ◯ tongue scraper
- ◯ hot towel scrub

- ◯ hot water bottle
- ◯ conscious breathing
- ◯ fresh air
- ◯ physical activity
- ◯ prayer/meditation
- ◯ meaningful connections

- ◯ loving work
- ◯ touch/massage
- ◯ laughter
- ◯ time to myself
- ◯ visualized my future
- ◯ quality sleep

high quality nourishment

water/hydrating liquids: _____

whole grains: _____

vegetables: _____

fruits: _____

healthy fats: _____

protein: _____

supplements: _____

how i felt today

mood: _____   digestion: _____

energy: _____   cravings: _____

today i appreciate myself for: _____

_____

choices that did not serve me or support me: _____

_____

today i added in or crowded out: _____

_____

loving thought before bed: _____

_____

morning intentions

date: _____

morning thoughts, feelings & intuitions: _____

_____

_____

_____

i am grateful for: _____

_____

_____

_____

goals for today:

◯ _____

◯ _____

◯ _____

action steps for each goal:

◯ _____ ◯ _____ ◯ _____

◯ _____ ◯ _____ ◯ _____

◯ _____ ◯ _____ ◯ _____

fun, relaxation & adventure for today:

◯ _____

◯ _____

◯ _____

evening reflections

○ morning intentions
○ home-cooked food (__x)
○ mindful eating
○ reduced one food
○ tongue scraper
○ hot towel scrub

○ hot water bottle
○ conscious breathing
○ fresh air
○ physical activity
○ prayer/meditation
○ meaningful connections

○ loving work
○ touch/massage
○ laughter
○ time to myself
○ visualized my future
○ quality sleep

high quality nourishment

water/hydrating liquids: _____

whole grains: _____

vegetables: _____

fruits: _____

healthy fats: _____

protein: _____

supplements: _____

how i felt today

mood: _____ digestion: _____

energy: _____ cravings: _____

today i appreciate myself for: _____

_____

choices that did not serve me or support me: _____

_____

today i added in or crowded out: _____

_____

loving thought before bed: _____

_____

morning intentions

date: _____

morning thoughts, feelings & intuitions: _____

_____

_____

_____

i am grateful for: _____

_____

_____

_____

goals for today:

○ _____

○ _____

○ _____

action steps for each goal:

○ _____ ○ _____ ○ _____

○ _____ ○ _____ ○ _____

○ _____ ○ _____ ○ _____

fun, relaxation & adventure for today:

○ _____

○ _____

○ _____

evening reflections

○ morning intentions
○ home-cooked food (__x)
○ mindful eating
○ reduced one food
○ tongue scraper
○ hot towel scrub

○ hot water bottle
○ conscious breathing
○ fresh air
○ physical activity
○ prayer/meditation
○ meaningful connections

○ loving work
○ touch/massage
○ laughter
○ time to myself
○ visualized my future
○ quality sleep

high quality nourishment

water/hydrating liquids: _____

whole grains: _____

vegetables: _____

fruits: _____

healthy fats: _____

protein: _____

supplements: _____

how i felt today

mood: _____ digestion: _____

energy: _____ cravings: _____

today i appreciate myself for: _____

_____

choices that did not serve me or support me: _____

_____

today i added in or crowded out: _____

_____

loving thought before bed: _____

_____

weekly check-in

dates: _____

what's new & good?

energy & vitality: _____
_____

chewing & digestion: _____
_____

cravings & addictions: _____
_____

hair & skin: _____
_____

mouth, teeth & tongue: _____
_____

body shape & weight: _____
_____

posture & breathing: _____
_____

mood & emotions: _____
_____

relating to others: _____
_____

about the week

most nourishing food: _____

_____

best primary food: _____

_____

special person i appreciate: _____

_____

biggest challenge: _____

_____

main health concern: _____

_____

greatest accomplishment: _____

_____

most fun i had: _____

_____

i got clear that i really want to: _____

_____

other thoughts: _____

_____

next week I plan to: _____

_____

guided exercise

my party

Without limitations on time, space or money,
describe the ultimate party you would throw to celebrate your life.

When and where would you have it?

Who would you invite?

What would the space, food and music be like?

When your life is in order you are transformed and heal.

Bernie Siegel, MD

morning intentions

date: _____

morning thoughts, feelings & intuitions: _____

_____

_____

_____

i am grateful for: _____

_____

_____

_____

goals for today:

○ _____

○ _____

○ _____

action steps for each goal:

○ _____ ○ _____ ○ _____

○ _____ ○ _____ ○ _____

○ _____ ○ _____ ○ _____

fun, relaxation & adventure for today:

○ _____

○ _____

○ _____

evening reflections

- ○ morning intentions
- ○ home-cooked food (__x)
- ○ mindful eating
- ○ reduced one food
- ○ tongue scraper
- ○ hot towel scrub

- ○ hot water bottle
- ○ conscious breathing
- ○ fresh air
- ○ physical activity
- ○ prayer/meditation
- ○ meaningful connections

- ○ loving work
- ○ touch/massage
- ○ laughter
- ○ time to myself
- ○ visualized my future
- ○ quality sleep

high quality nourishment

water/hydrating liquids: _____

whole grains: _____

vegetables: _____

fruits: _____

healthy fats: _____

protein: _____

supplements: _____

how i felt today

mood: _____ digestion: _____

energy: _____ cravings: _____

today i appreciate myself for: _____

_____

choices that did not serve me or support me: _____

_____

today i added in or crowded out: _____

_____

loving thought before bed: _____

_____

morning intentions

date: _____

morning thoughts, feelings & intuitions: _____

_____

_____

_____

i am grateful for: _____

_____

_____

_____

goals for today:

○ _____

○ _____

○ _____

action steps for each goal:

○ _____ ○ _____ ○ _____

○ _____ ○ _____ ○ _____

○ _____ ○ _____ ○ _____

fun, relaxation & adventure for today:

○ _____

○ _____

○ _____

evening reflections

- ⃝ morning intentions
- ⃝ home-cooked food (__x)
- ⃝ mindful eating
- ⃝ reduced one food
- ⃝ tongue scraper
- ⃝ hot towel scrub

- ⃝ hot water bottle
- ⃝ conscious breathing
- ⃝ fresh air
- ⃝ physical activity
- ⃝ prayer/meditation
- ⃝ meaningful connections

- ⃝ loving work
- ⃝ touch/massage
- ⃝ laughter
- ⃝ time to myself
- ⃝ visualized my future
- ⃝ quality sleep

high quality nourishment

water/hydrating liquids: _____

whole grains: _____

vegetables: _____

fruits: _____

healthy fats: _____

protein: _____

supplements: _____

how i felt today

mood: _____   digestion: _____

energy: _____   cravings: _____

today i appreciate myself for: _____

_____

choices that did not serve me or support me: _____

_____

today i added in or crowded out: _____

_____

loving thought before bed: _____

_____

morning intentions

date: _____

morning thoughts, feelings & intuitions: _____

_____

_____

_____

i am grateful for: _____

_____

_____

_____

goals for today:

◯ _____

◯ _____

◯ _____

action steps for each goal:

◯ _____ ◯ _____ ◯ _____

◯ _____ ◯ _____ ◯ _____

◯ _____ ◯ _____ ◯ _____

fun, relaxation & adventure for today:

◯ _____

◯ _____

◯ _____

evening reflections

- ○ morning intentions
- ○ home-cooked food (__x)
- ○ mindful eating
- ○ reduced one food
- ○ tongue scraper
- ○ hot towel scrub

- ○ hot water bottle
- ○ conscious breathing
- ○ fresh air
- ○ physical activity
- ○ prayer/meditation
- ○ meaningful connections

- ○ loving work
- ○ touch/massage
- ○ laughter
- ○ time to myself
- ○ visualized my future
- ○ quality sleep

high quality nourishment

water/hydrating liquids: _____

whole grains: _____

vegetables: _____

fruits: _____

healthy fats: _____

protein: _____

supplements: _____

how i felt today

mood: _____ digestion: _____

energy: _____ cravings: _____

today i appreciate myself for: _____

_____

choices that did not serve me or support me: _____

_____

today i added in or crowded out: _____

_____

loving thought before bed: _____

_____

morning intentions

date: _____

morning thoughts, feelings & intuitions: _____

_____

_____

_____

i am grateful for: _____

_____

_____

_____

goals for today:

○ _____

○ _____

○ _____

action steps for each goal:

○ _____   ○ _____   ○ _____

○ _____   ○ _____   ○ _____

○ _____   ○ _____   ○ _____

fun, relaxation & adventure for today:

○ _____

○ _____

○ _____

evening reflections

○ morning intentions
○ home-cooked food (__x)
○ mindful eating
○ reduced one food
○ tongue scraper
○ hot towel scrub

○ hot water bottle
○ conscious breathing
○ fresh air
○ physical activity
○ prayer/meditation
○ meaningful connections

○ loving work
○ touch/massage
○ laughter
○ time to myself
○ visualized my future
○ quality sleep

high quality nourishment

water/hydrating liquids: _____

whole grains: _____

vegetables: _____

fruits: _____

healthy fats: _____

protein: _____

supplements: _____

how i felt today

mood: _____ digestion: _____

energy: _____ cravings: _____

today i appreciate myself for: _____

_____

choices that did not serve me or support me: _____

_____

today i added in or crowded out: _____

_____

loving thought before bed: _____

_____

morning intentions

date: _____

morning thoughts, feelings & intuitions: _____

_____

_____

_____

i am grateful for: _____

_____

_____

_____

goals for today:

◯ _____

◯ _____

◯ _____

action steps for each goal:

◯ _____ ◯ _____ ◯ _____

◯ _____ ◯ _____ ◯ _____

◯ _____ ◯ _____ ◯ _____

fun, relaxation & adventure for today:

◯ _____

◯ _____

◯ _____

evening reflections

○ morning intentions   ○ hot water bottle   ○ loving work
○ home-cooked food (__x)   ○ conscious breathing   ○ touch/massage
○ mindful eating   ○ fresh air   ○ laughter
○ reduced one food   ○ physical activity   ○ time to myself
○ tongue scraper   ○ prayer/meditation   ○ visualized my future
○ hot towel scrub   ○ meaningful connections   ○ quality sleep

high quality nourishment

water/hydrating liquids: _____

whole grains: _____

vegetables: _____

fruits: _____

healthy fats: _____

protein: _____

supplements: _____

how i felt today

mood: _____   digestion: _____

energy: _____   cravings: _____

today i appreciate myself for: _____

_____

choices that did not serve me or support me: _____

_____

today i added in or crowded out: _____

_____

loving thought before bed: _____

_____

morning intentions

date: _____

morning thoughts, feelings & intuitions: _____

_____

_____

_____

i am grateful for: _____

_____

_____

_____

goals for today:

○ _____

○ _____

○ _____

action steps for each goal:

○ _____ ○ _____ ○ _____

○ _____ ○ _____ ○ _____

○ _____ ○ _____ ○ _____

fun, relaxation & adventure for today:

○ _____

○ _____

○ _____

evening reflections

- ○ morning intentions
- ○ home-cooked food (__x)
- ○ mindful eating
- ○ reduced one food
- ○ tongue scraper
- ○ hot towel scrub

- ○ hot water bottle
- ○ conscious breathing
- ○ fresh air
- ○ physical activity
- ○ prayer/meditation
- ○ meaningful connections

- ○ loving work
- ○ touch/massage
- ○ laughter
- ○ time to myself
- ○ visualized my future
- ○ quality sleep

high quality nourishment

water/hydrating liquids: _____

whole grains: _____

vegetables: _____

fruits: _____

healthy fats: _____

protein: _____

supplements: _____

how i felt today

mood: _____   digestion: _____

energy: _____   cravings: _____

today i appreciate myself for: _____

_____

choices that did not serve me or support me: _____

_____

today i added in or crowded out: _____

_____

loving thought before bed: _____

_____

morning intentions

date: _____

morning thoughts, feelings & intuitions: _____

_____

_____

_____

i am grateful for: _____

_____

_____

_____

goals for today:

◯ _____

◯ _____

◯ _____

action steps for each goal:

◯ _____ ◯ _____ ◯ _____

◯ _____ ◯ _____ ◯ _____

◯ _____ ◯ _____ ◯ _____

fun, relaxation & adventure for today:

◯ _____

◯ _____

◯ _____

evening reflections

○ morning intentions
○ home-cooked food (__x)
○ mindful eating
○ reduced one food
○ tongue scraper
○ hot towel scrub

○ hot water bottle
○ conscious breathing
○ fresh air
○ physical activity
○ prayer/meditation
○ meaningful connections

○ loving work
○ touch/massage
○ laughter
○ time to myself
○ visualized my future
○ quality sleep

high quality nourishment

water/hydrating liquids: _____

whole grains: _____

vegetables: _____

fruits: _____

healthy fats: _____

protein: _____

supplements: _____

how i felt today

mood: _____ digestion: _____

energy: _____ cravings: _____

today i appreciate myself for: _____

_____

choices that did not serve me or support me: _____

_____

today i added in or crowded out: _____

_____

loving thought before bed: _____

_____

weekly check-in

dates: _____

what's new & good?

energy & vitality: _____
_____

chewing & digestion: _____
_____

cravings & addictions: _____
_____

hair & skin: _____
_____

mouth, teeth & tongue: _____
_____

body shape & weight: _____
_____

posture & breathing: _____
_____

mood & emotions: _____
_____

relating to others: _____
_____

about the week

most nourishing food: _____

_____

best primary food: _____

_____

special person i appreciate: _____

_____

biggest challenge: _____

_____

main health concern: _____

_____

greatest accomplishment: _____

_____

most fun i had: _____

_____

i got clear that i really want to: _____

_____

other thoughts: _____

_____

next week I plan to: _____

_____

guided exercise

my contribution

Using all your talent and passion,
what is one big contribution you would like to make to the world?
Describe it in detail.

Who would be touched by your contribution and how would it affect them?

How would it feel to make this contribution?

We must ask ourselves, if we wish to be healthy, what for?
To what use will we put our health?

Annemarie Colbin, PhD

morning intentions

date: _____

morning thoughts, feelings & intuitions: _____

_____

_____

_____

i am grateful for: _____

_____

_____

_____

goals for today:

○ _____

○ _____

○ _____

action steps for each goal:

○ _____ ○ _____ ○ _____

○ _____ ○ _____ ○ _____

○ _____ ○ _____ ○ _____

fun, relaxation & adventure for today:

○ _____

○ _____

○ _____

evening reflections

○ morning intentions
○ home-cooked food (__x)
○ mindful eating
○ reduced one food
○ tongue scraper
○ hot towel scrub

○ hot water bottle
○ conscious breathing
○ fresh air
○ physical activity
○ prayer/meditation
○ meaningful connections

○ loving work
○ touch/massage
○ laughter
○ time to myself
○ visualized my future
○ quality sleep

high quality nourishment

water/hydrating liquids: _____

whole grains: _____

vegetables: _____

fruits: _____

healthy fats: _____

protein: _____

supplements: _____

how i felt today

mood: _____   digestion: _____

energy: _____   cravings: _____

today i appreciate myself for: _____

_____

choices that did not serve me or support me: _____

_____

today i added in or crowded out: _____

_____

loving thought before bed: _____

_____

morning intentions

date: _____

morning thoughts, feelings & intuitions: _____

_____

_____

_____

i am grateful for: _____

_____

_____

_____

goals for today:

○ _____

○ _____

○ _____

action steps for each goal:

○ _____ ○ _____ ○ _____

○ _____ ○ _____ ○ _____

○ _____ ○ _____ ○ _____

fun, relaxation & adventure for today:

○ _____

○ _____

○ _____

evening reflections

- ○ morning intentions
- ○ home-cooked food (__x)
- ○ mindful eating
- ○ reduced one food
- ○ tongue scraper
- ○ hot towel scrub

- ○ hot water bottle
- ○ conscious breathing
- ○ fresh air
- ○ physical activity
- ○ prayer/meditation
- ○ meaningful connections

- ○ loving work
- ○ touch/massage
- ○ laughter
- ○ time to myself
- ○ visualized my future
- ○ quality sleep

high quality nourishment

water/hydrating liquids: _____

whole grains: _____

vegetables: _____

fruits: _____

healthy fats: _____

protein: _____

supplements: _____

how i felt today

mood: _____ digestion: _____

energy: _____ cravings: _____

today i appreciate myself for: _____

_____

choices that did not serve me or support me: _____

_____

today i added in or crowded out: _____

_____

loving thought before bed: _____

_____

morning intentions

date: _____

morning thoughts, feelings & intuitions: _____

_____

_____

_____

i am grateful for: _____

_____

_____

_____

goals for today:

○ _____

○ _____

○ _____

action steps for each goal:

○ _____ ○ _____ ○ _____

○ _____ ○ _____ ○ _____

○ _____ ○ _____ ○ _____

fun, relaxation & adventure for today:

○ _____

○ _____

○ _____

evening reflections

- ○ morning intentions
- ○ home-cooked food (__x)
- ○ mindful eating
- ○ reduced one food
- ○ tongue scraper
- ○ hot towel scrub

- ○ hot water bottle
- ○ conscious breathing
- ○ fresh air
- ○ physical activity
- ○ prayer/meditation
- ○ meaningful connections

- ○ loving work
- ○ touch/massage
- ○ laughter
- ○ time to myself
- ○ visualized my future
- ○ quality sleep

high quality nourishment

water/hydrating liquids: _____

whole grains: _____

vegetables: _____

fruits: _____

healthy fats: _____

protein: _____

supplements: _____

how i felt today

mood: _____   digestion: _____

energy: _____   cravings: _____

today i appreciate myself for: _____

_____

choices that did not serve me or support me: _____

_____

today i added in or crowded out: _____

_____

loving thought before bed: _____

_____

morning intentions

date: _____

morning thoughts, feelings & intuitions: _____
_____
_____
_____

i am grateful for: _____
_____
_____
_____

goals for today:

○ _____
○ _____
○ _____

action steps for each goal:

○ _____ ○ _____ ○ _____
○ _____ ○ _____ ○ _____
○ _____ ○ _____ ○ _____

fun, relaxation & adventure for today:

○ _____
○ _____
○ _____

evening reflections

○ morning intentions   ○ hot water bottle   ○ loving work
○ home-cooked food (__x)   ○ conscious breathing   ○ touch/massage
○ mindful eating   ○ fresh air   ○ laughter
○ reduced one food   ○ physical activity   ○ time to myself
○ tongue scraper   ○ prayer/meditation   ○ visualized my future
○ hot towel scrub   ○ meaningful connections   ○ quality sleep

high quality nourishment

water/hydrating liquids: _____

whole grains: _____

vegetables: _____

fruits: _____

healthy fats: _____

protein: _____

supplements: _____

how i felt today

mood: _____ digestion: _____

energy: _____ cravings: _____

today i appreciate myself for: _____

_____

choices that did not serve me or support me: _____

_____

today i added in or crowded out: _____

_____

loving thought before bed: _____

_____

morning intentions

date: _____

morning thoughts, feelings & intuitions: _____

_____

_____

_____

i am grateful for: _____

_____

_____

_____

goals for today:

◯ _____

◯ _____

◯ _____

action steps for each goal:

◯ _____ ◯ _____ ◯ _____

◯ _____ ◯ _____ ◯ _____

◯ _____ ◯ _____ ◯ _____

fun, relaxation & adventure for today:

◯ _____

◯ _____

◯ _____

evening reflections

- ○ morning intentions
- ○ home-cooked food (__x)
- ○ mindful eating
- ○ reduced one food
- ○ tongue scraper
- ○ hot towel scrub

- ○ hot water bottle
- ○ conscious breathing
- ○ fresh air
- ○ physical activity
- ○ prayer/meditation
- ○ meaningful connections

- ○ loving work
- ○ touch/massage
- ○ laughter
- ○ time to myself
- ○ visualized my future
- ○ quality sleep

high quality nourishment

water/hydrating liquids: _____

whole grains: _____

vegetables: _____

fruits: _____

healthy fats: _____

protein: _____

supplements: _____

how i felt today

mood: _____ digestion: _____

energy: _____ cravings: _____

today i appreciate myself for: _____

_____

choices that did not serve me or support me: _____

_____

today i added in or crowded out: _____

_____

loving thought before bed: _____

_____

morning intentions

date: _____

morning thoughts, feelings & intuitions: _____

_____

_____

_____

i am grateful for: _____

_____

_____

_____

goals for today:

○ _____

○ _____

○ _____

action steps for each goal:

○ _____ ○ _____ ○ _____

○ _____ ○ _____ ○ _____

○ _____ ○ _____ ○ _____

fun, relaxation & adventure for today:

○ _____

○ _____

○ _____

evening reflections

- ○ morning intentions
- ○ home-cooked food (__x)
- ○ mindful eating
- ○ reduced one food
- ○ tongue scraper
- ○ hot towel scrub

- ○ hot water bottle
- ○ conscious breathing
- ○ fresh air
- ○ physical activity
- ○ prayer/meditation
- ○ meaningful connections

- ○ loving work
- ○ touch/massage
- ○ laughter
- ○ time to myself
- ○ visualized my future
- ○ quality sleep

high quality nourishment

water/hydrating liquids: _____

whole grains: _____

vegetables: _____

fruits: _____

healthy fats: _____

protein: _____

supplements: _____

how i felt today

mood: _____   digestion: _____

energy: _____   cravings: _____

today i appreciate myself for: _____

_____

choices that did not serve me or support me: _____

_____

today i added in or crowded out: _____

_____

loving thought before bed: _____

_____

morning intentions

date: _____

morning thoughts, feelings & intuitions: _____

_____

_____

_____

i am grateful for: _____

_____

_____

_____

goals for today:

○ _____

○ _____

○ _____

action steps for each goal:

○ _____ ○ _____ ○ _____

○ _____ ○ _____ ○ _____

○ _____ ○ _____ ○ _____

fun, relaxation & adventure for today:

○ _____

○ _____

○ _____

evening reflections

- ○ morning intentions
- ○ home-cooked food (__x)
- ○ mindful eating
- ○ reduced one food
- ○ tongue scraper
- ○ hot towel scrub

- ○ hot water bottle
- ○ conscious breathing
- ○ fresh air
- ○ physical activity
- ○ prayer/meditation
- ○ meaningful connections

- ○ loving work
- ○ touch/massage
- ○ laughter
- ○ time to myself
- ○ visualized my future
- ○ quality sleep

high quality nourishment

water/hydrating liquids: _____

whole grains: _____

vegetables: _____

fruits: _____

healthy fats: _____

protein: _____

supplements: _____

how i felt today

mood: _____ digestion: _____

energy: _____ cravings: _____

today i appreciate myself for: _____

_____

choices that did not serve me or support me: _____

_____

today i added in or crowded out: _____

_____

loving thought before bed: _____

_____

month three progress

dates: _____

what's changed this month?

food & cooking: _____

_____

_____

self-care: _____

_____

_____

physical health: _____

_____

_____

main health concern: _____

_____

_____

habits, cravings & addictions: _____

_____

_____

moods, thoughts & feelings: _____

_____

_____

primary food progress

career: _____

_____

relationships: _____

_____

physical activity: _____

_____

spirituality: _____

_____

creativity: _____

_____

fun, relaxation & adventure: _____

_____

other accomplishments: _____

_____

_____

_____

_____

_____

_____

Changing our diet is more powerful than most of us have imagined.

Neal Barnard, MD

circle of life

Congratulations on completing your journal! Use this final Circle of Life to see how far you've come since you started. You will probably notice that your circle is larger and more balanced, going more in the direction of ultimate happiness in all areas. You might also see some areas that still need attention. That's okay too. Now that you have learned the skills you need to create personal wellness, we encourage you to keep going. Imagine how balanced and fulfilling your life would be if you took care of yourself this way for 3 more months, 1 year, 5 years or 10 years.

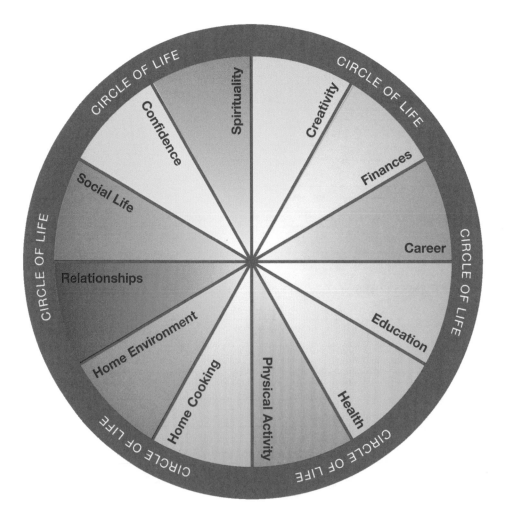

wish list

Looking at your Circle of Life and your past wish lists, what other desires do you want to fulfill in your future? As you continue to eat well, care for your body and focus on your hopes and dreams, you will find more and more of your wishes coming true. We've noticed that this process often speeds up after the first 3 months, once physical health is much better. As you go forward, regular use of wish lists will keep you connected to your authentic desires and help you create the amazing life you were born to live.

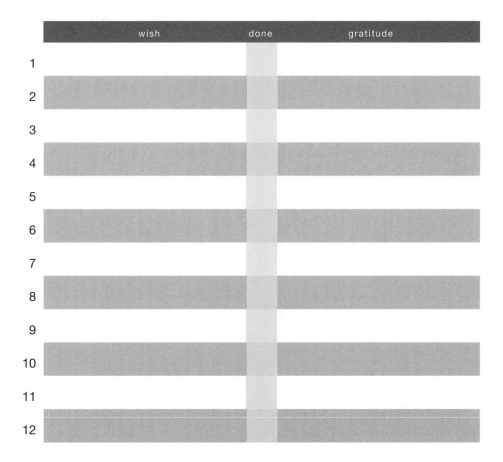

	wish	done	gratitude
1			
2			
3			
4			
5			
6			
7			
8			
9			
10			
11			
12			

Eat well, be active, don't smoke, get some sleep,
find somebody to love who preferably loves you
back, and try not to stress out excessively.

David Katz, MD

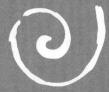

glossary

add in/crowd out: Most diets give people a list of foods to avoid and foods to eat. This is why so many people are turned off by diets. We have found a more effective method we call "crowding out." This entails adding in health-promoting foods and beverages, such as vegetables, whole grains, healthy fats, high-quality protein and water, which leaves less room for—or crowds out—unhealthy foods.

conscious breathing: When busy and stressed, most people breathe shallowly, depriving their bodies of necessary oxygen. By breathing slowly and deeply, you allow your body to relax and your mind to focus.

cravings: Cravings are not a problem—they are your body's way of communicating to you what it needs. For example, sugar cravings may indicate you need more water, relaxation or love. Salty cravings may mean you need more minerals or nutrient-dense foods. As you deconstruct and respond to your cravings, your body will come into balance, and the cravings will fade.

healthy fats: Not all fats are bad. Healthy oils include coconut, extra virgin olive, sesame or walnut. Healthy fats can be found in natural organic butter, whole nuts and seeds, nut butters, avocados, wild salmon and organic eggs. Try having small quantities of healthy fat daily.

hot towel scrub: Take a washcloth, wet it with hot water, wring it out and then rub your entire body for five to 10 minutes. This practice calms body and mind, supports detoxification and helps you build a loving connection with your body.

hot water bottle: At bedtime, or anytime comfort is needed, place an old-fashioned hot water bottle on your belly for 15 to 20 minutes. The heat brings energy and blood circulation to digestive organs, plus creates a sense of comfort and relaxation.

hydrating liquids: Herbal tea, soup and natural juice all help hydrate the body, although not as much as water. Caffeinated drinks don't count because they are dehydrating. Experiment to see which liquids help you feel balanced and hydrated.

meaningful connections: Nurture and make time for your high-quality relationships, whether with family, friends or co-workers. Having a community that supports you and your goals is very important for a satisfying life.

mindful eating: To improve digestion and nutrient absorption, give your meals your full attention. Notice the flavors, textures and colors of your food and chew thoroughly. When possible, eat in a quiet place away from the computer and TV.

primary food: We call anything in your life that nourishes you, but does not come on a plate, primary food. The important primary food areas are:
> Career: Find work you love or find a way to love the work you have.
> Relationships: Have healthy relationships that support you.
> Physical Activity: Find a form of movement you enjoy and do it regularly.
> Spirituality: Develop a spiritual practice that fits your beliefs and gives depth and meaning to your life.

protein: Protein is good for us. Protein requirements differ dramatically from person to person. Experiment with reducing or increasing your amount of protein, and try different types. Some people need animal food, while others thrive on vegetarian protein sources like grain and bean combinations or natural soy products. Listen to your body to find out what is best for you. There is no right or wrong here.

reduce one food: There is no dietary practice that is right for everyone, but you will most likely get healthier if you have less meat, dairy, sugar, chemicalized artificial junk foods, coffee, alcohol and tobacco.

tongue scraper: This simple, thin, u-shaped piece of stainless steel with a safely blunted edge removes gunk from the surface of your tongue. It helps with cravings and bad breath, and also improves your ability to taste food.

touch/massage: People thrive on human touch, warmth and intimacy. Figure out how to have more positive touch in your life. Choose any type that works for you, such as hugs from friends, sex with a partner or massage from a licensed body worker.

visualize your future: Put time and energy into imagining what you want your life to look and feel like. The clearer your intentions are, the more likely it is that the future you desire will happen.

whole grains: Grains in their whole, natural form are generally healthier than refined grain foods like breads, pastas and pastries. Whole grains digest slowly, provide sustained energy and supply needed fiber and nutrients. Some common whole grains are brown rice, quinoa, buckwheat, oats and millet.

The foods and primary foods recommended in this journal are described in more detail in our book *Integrative Nutrition: The Future of Nutrition,* by Joshua Rosenthal.

The more we live in balance and respect
nature and ourselves,
the more likely we are to be in the right place
at the right time, all the time.

Joshua Rosenthal, MScEd

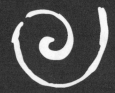

about integrative nutrition

After taking great care of yourself for the past 3 months, you are probably feeling happier and healthier than ever before. We invite you to use this newfound energy to create what you really want in your life. You have unlimited potential. As a healthy, happy person you can make a positive difference in the world, while living the life you desire.

If helping others achieve a high level of health and happiness interests you, we invite you to check out our school. Integrative Nutrition provides the latest, most cutting-edge information about nutrition and lifestyle. Our students receive a life-changing education within a nurturing environment. We teach them to become certified health coaches and take an active role in changing the health and happiness of others.

www.integrativenutrition.com

notes

notes

notes

notes

notes

notes